THE PRACTICAL GUIDE TO MEDICAL ETHICS AND LAW

Second Edition

Chloë-Maryse Baxter
BSc(Hons) MB ChB (Manchester) MHPE (Maastricht)

Mark G Brennan
BA(Hons) (Surrey) MA (London) AKC DHMSA ILTM FRIPH

Yvette G M Coldicott
BSc(Hons) MB ChB (Bristol)

Maaike Möller
BSc(Hons) MB ChB (Bristol)

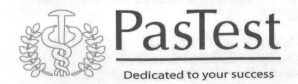

Dedicated to your success

© 2005 PASTEST LTD
Egerton Court
Parkgate Estate
Knutsford
Cheshire
WA16 8DX

Telephone: 01565 752000

First published 2002
Reprinted 2003
Second edition 2005

ISBN: 1 904627 31 5

A catalogue record for this book is available from the British Library.

The information contained within this book was obtained by the author from reliable sources. However, while every effort has been made to ensure its accuracy, no responsibility for loss, damage or injury occasioned to any person acting or refraining from action as a result of information contained herein can be accepted by the publishers or author.

PasTest Revision Books and Intensive Courses

PasTest has been established in the field of postgraduate medical education since 1972, providing revision books and intensive study courses for doctors preparing for their professional examinations.

Books and courses are available for the following specialties:
MRCGP, MRCP Parts 1 and 2, MRCPCH Parts 1 and 2, MRCPsych, MRCS, MRCOG Parts 1 and 2, DRCOG, DCH, FRCA, PLAB Parts 1 and 2.

For further details contact:
PasTest, Freepost, Knutsford, Cheshire WA16 7BR

Tel: 01565 752000
www.pastest.co.uk

Fax: 01565 650264
enquiries@pastest.co.uk

Typeset by Type Study, Scarborough, North Yorkshire
Printed and bound by MPG Books, Bodmin, Cornwall

.LEY

THE PRACTICAL GUIDE TO
MEDICAL ETHICS AND LAW

Second Edition

THE PRACTICAL GUIDE TO
MEDICAL ETHICS AND LAW

PasTest

Dedicated to your success

CONTENTS

ABOUT THE AUTHORS

Dr Chloë-Maryse Baxter
BSc(Hons) MB ChB with European Studies (Manchester)
MHPE (Maastricht)

Chloë Baxter graduated from Manchester Medical School in 2001, MB ChB with European Studies, having also obtained an intercalated BSc in Health Care Ethics and Law. She was a pre-registration house officer in Edinburgh before heading to Sydney, Australia, to continue her clinical training in paediatrics. During this time, she studied for the Masters degree in Health Professions Education at Maastricht University in the Netherlands and completed this in 2003.

Mark G Brennan
BA(Hons) (Surrey) MA (London) AKC DHMSA ILTM FRIPH

Mark Brennan obtained his MA in Medical Ethics and Law at King's College London in 1991. He is currently head of division and senior lecturer in clinical education in the Kent Institute of Medicine and Health Sciences at the University of Kent. He was formerly a lecturer in medical and dental education and Education Tutor for Wales at Cardiff University, a visiting senior lecturer in medical ethics at the Royal College of Surgeons in Ireland and at Trinity College Dublin, and a lecturer in medical ethics and honorary research fellow at Bristol University's Centre for Ethics in Medicine. He has been the education adviser to the Medical Defence Union in the UK since 1996, with whom he has established a programme of ethics workshops for qualified doctors.

Dr Yvette G M Colidcott
BSc(Hons) MB ChB (Bristol)

Yvette Coldicott graduated from Bristol University in 2002, where she also obtained an intercalated BSc in Bioethics. She was a pre-registration house officer at Bristol Royal Infirmary and is now a senior house officer in Medicine. She plans to continue her clinical career in anaesthetics.

Dr Maaike Möller
BSc(Hons) MB ChB (Bristol)

Maaike Möller graduated from Bristol University in 2004 and was a pre-registration house officer in Cheltenham at the time of writing. She did an intercalated BSc in Bioethics and has retained an interest in the subject ever since. Her other particular interest is international medicine and she intends to work in the developing world in the future. She is currently a senior house officer in Homerton Hospital, London.

Acknowledgements

We dedicate this book to our families and friends; those who taught each of us about medical ethics and law in practice, and those whom we now teach; our patients and colleagues in healthcare and to our team of international contributors, with thanks for all their support, encouragement and inspiration.

PRINCIPAL CONTRIBUTORS

Deborah Bowman BA MA
Deborah Bowman is Senior Lecturer in Medical Ethics and Law at St George's Hospital Medical School, where she is also Personal and Professional Development Theme Lead on the Graduate Entry Programme in Medicine. She is a member of the Unrelated Live Transplant Regulatory Authority.

Dr Richard Huxtable LLB(Hons) (Nottingham) MA (Sheffield) PhD (Bristol)
Richard Huxtable is Lecturer in Medical Law and Ethics at the Centre for Ethics in Medicine at Bristol University. He teaches health professionals and students of Medicine and Law, and directs the intercalated BSc in Bioethics and MSc in Health Care Ethics.

Professor Bill Shannon MD FRCGP MICGP
Bill Shannon is Head of Department of General Practice and Family Medicine at the Royal College of Surgeons in Ireland Medical School in Dublin, RCSI Academic Lead at Penang Medical College in Malaysia, and Tutor and Co-ordinator of the Family Practice Residency Programme in Bahrain. He teaches medical ethics and law at both undergraduate and postgraduate levels.

CONTRIBUTORS:

Dr Shrilla Banerjee, London, England
Dr Jamiu Busari, Curaçao, Netherlands Antilles
Dr Kosta Calligeros, Edinburgh, Scotland
Mr Michael Carmont, Oswestry, England
Dr Stephen Child, Auckland, New Zealand
Dr Alejandro Cragno, Buenos Aires, Argentina
Prof Michel Gillet, Lausanne, Switzerland
Dr Nermin Halkic, Lausanne, Switzerland
Dr David Joseph, Sydney, Australia
Prof Mitchell Levy, Providence (RI), USA
Dr Vassilis Lykomitros, Athens, Greece
Dr Dhruv Mankad, Nasik, India
Prof Marcellina Mian, Toronto, Canada
Dr Peter Mills, London, England
Dr Elizabeth Morris, Edinburgh, Scotland
Dr Emma Nelson, Dublin, Ireland
Mr Jonathan Osborn, Chicago (IL), USA
Dr Christina Panteli, Thessaloniki, Greece
Dr Sophie Park, London, England
Prof Graham Ramsay, Maastricht, The Netherlands
Prof Peter Rosen, San Diego (CA), USA
Dr Guy Routh, Cheltenham, England
Dr Francesca Rubulotta, Providence (RI), USA
Dr Joan Saary, Toronto, Canada
Dr Adrian Sutton, Manchester, England
Dr Andy Swain, Palmerston North, New Zealand
Dr Bob Taylor, Belfast, Northern Ireland
Dr Antony Toft, Edinburgh, Scotland
Dr Hamish Wallace, Edinburgh, Scotland
Associate Prof Merrilyn Walton, Sydney, Australia
Prof Valerie Wass, Manchester, England

PERMISSIONS:

PasTest would like to thank the following for allowing material to be used in this book:

British Medical Association
General Medical Council

FOREWORD

Professor Jill Gordon

MB BS (University of Sydney), BA (University of Newcastle), MPsychMed (University of New South Wales), PhD (University of Newcastle), FRACGP

Director, Centre for Medical Humanities, University of Sydney

In 1908, John Dewey and James Tufts wrote, *'the (moral) theorist . . . must take his departure from the problems which men actually meet in their own conduct. He may define and refine these; he may divide and systematise; he may abstract the problems from their concrete contexts in individual lives . . . but if he gets away from them, he is talking about something his own brain has invented, not about moral realities.'*

It's a great pleasure to see that this second edition of *The Practical Guide to Medical Ethics and Law* has retained this central characteristic of dealing with the real problems that confront us. You won't find all of these ethical dilemmas on the front page of the newspaper or in the television news, but they affect more lives than most of the exotic issues in the headlines. Rather than portraying doctors as white knights or black demons, they capture the complexities of life as a medical student or junior doctor.

The problem inherent in any dilemma can be found in the definition of the word itself. A *di-lemma* is concerned with two valid but opposed propositions. Because neither proposition can be totally invalidated, a dilemma can never be fully resolved. The problem of competing rights, such as the rights of the pregnant woman and of her unborn baby, is a classic example.

Day-to-day practice is full of simple but important dilemmas – whether or not to provide a patient with certain information, to recommend a test or to use a particular treatment. Even in the course of making 'ordinary' clinical decisions, thoughtful doctors know that they might have made another, different choice. We cannot know where that other decision would have led us and our patients, and we cannot be certain of having done the greatest good and the least possible harm in every case, no matter how hard we try. Lawyers operate with the benefit of the 'retrospectoscope', but doctors cope with the untidiness of the 'here and now'.

Doctors can be tempted to seek a greater sense of certainty. They can:

(a) fail to notice that an ethical dilemmas exists,
(b) treat each dilemma as if it were simply a debate to be won or lost, or
(c) behave as though ethical dilemmas can be resolved by technical means – that given 'enough science', the right answer will eventually reveal itself.

The real-life examples in this book illustrate why it is that these responses are unsatisfactory. Doctors who fail to notice the presence of ethical dilemmas also fail to grow, both personally and professionally. Doctors who think dilemmas can be 'won or lost' like debates deny the subtlety and complexity of their human experience. The reductionists take the most frightening path of all, by failing to understand that 'value-free' science has led to some of the worst ethical abuses in human history.

By contrast, the contributors to this book show that they know just how uncertain and messy medicine can be. Medical students and junior doctors who wonder if they are the only people who have not yet found the One Right Answer can rest assured that dilemmas are just that – unresolved questions that nevertheless demand action and practical responses.

Paradoxically, the experiences described in this book do not lead to a position of ethical nihilism. They demonstrate, among other things, the importance of virtue as a guide to action. William Osler was drawn to the conclusion that, *'the greatest therapeutic gifts are kindness, human understanding, sympathy and common sense (which) in a continually changing scientific world . . . remain permanently desirable attributes.'*

Congratulations to Chloë Baxter, Mark Brennan, Yvette Coldicott and Maaike Möller for gathering these stories together in this new edition. They have donated their wisdom, expertise and experience, both medical and ethical, to create a 'therapeutic gift' for their readership.

ABBREVIATIONS

A&E	accident and emergency department
AIDS	acquired immune deficiency syndrome
ATN	acute tubular necrosis
AVR	aortic valve replacement
BAL	broncho-alveolar lavage
BMA	British Medical Association
BMI	body mass index
BSc	Bachelor of Science
CMO	comfort measures only
COPE	Committee On Publication Ethics
CT	computed tomography
DNAR	do not attempt resuscitation
DVLA	Driver and Vehicle Licensing Authority
ECHR	European Court of Human Rights
ECT	electro-convulsive therapy
EU	European Union
FBC	full blood count
GCS	Glasgow Coma Scale
GMC	General Medical Council
GP	general practitioner
HFEA	Human Fertilisation and Embryology Authority
HIV	human immunodeficiency virus
ICU	intensive care unit
IUD	intra-uterine device
IVF	in vitro fertilisation
MCQ	multiple choice question
MHAC	Mental Health Act Commission
MHRT	mental health review tribunal
MMR	measles, mumps and rubella
NHS	National Health Service
NICE	National Institute for Clinical Excellence
ODP	operating department practitioner
OSCE	Objective Structured Clinical Examination
PIGD	pre-implantation genetic diagnosis
PLAB	Professional and Linguistic Assessment Board (test)
PSA	prostate-specific antigen
QALY	quality-adjusted life-year

SHO   senior house officer
SpR   specialist registrar
SSC   student selected component
SSM   special study module
UKRC   United Kingdom Resuscitation Council
ULTRA   Unrelated Live Transplant Regulatory Authority
UTI   urinary tract infection

Chapter One
INTRODUCTION

Welcome to The Practical Guide to Medical Ethics and Law! Although the book is primarily intended for doctors and medical students, it will also be of interest to other health professionals, to teachers of medical ethics and law, and other medical teachers and medical scientists, to those studying bioscience and other disciplines, and to those who have an interest in the subject.

While preparing this second edition of the book we have responded to feedback from readers, as well as from our colleagues and students. A considerable amount of new material has been added. The first edition was aimed at medical students and junior doctors. However, it has become clear that our readership is broader than we had first envisaged and includes more senior doctors too, as well as teachers of ethics and law and others. We have therefore included a new chapter on how to teach medical ethics and law.

By their very nature, ethics and law are dynamic subjects and changing all the time. We have sought to include recent legislation and other developments, updating the original text where appropriate and adding new cases which illustrate some of the current advances in medicine as well as the concomitant ethical and legal challenges. The writing team has been expanded and now comprises four authors and three principal contributors, representing practising clinicians, medical ethicists and qualified lawyers. We are all involved in teaching the theory and practice of medical ethics and law.

The main body of the book is made up of case studies. Studying clinical cases is the most efficient way to learn anything in medicine, and ethics and law is no exception. The cases in Chapter 5 have been worked out for you, giving a clear structure for approaching ethical and legal problems. All of these cases are based on real-life situations either known to the authors or described to us by friends and colleagues. Mostly, they are a composite of incidents and events involving a range of patients, doctors and medical students in both hospital and primary care settings. Details of both patients and doctors have been altered to ensure anonymity and protect confidentiality where appropriate. You can use these cases in a variety of ways:

- You can work through them on your own, in stages.
- You can work through them with others in a group. This is the most efficient way of covering the issues because you can discuss and debate various points of view together. Working in a group is obviously good practice for working life as a doctor, because it requires you to tolerate and accept the existence of alternative views,

and yet justify and defend your arguments to yourself and others. It is also good practice for exams.

■ You can read through them as a revision exercise. Key revision points are indicated so that you can easily spot them, and at the end of each case there is a summary.

■ Teachers may choose to use the cases as triggers for a discussion.

The cases in Chapter 6 come from doctors all over the world. They are real-life examples of ethico-legal dilemmas in clinical practice, which illustrate that even the most experienced clinicians can find such dilemmas difficult to deal with. Again, patient details have been altered to maintain confidentiality.

SO WHY STUDY MEDICAL ETHICS AND LAW?

A young vet from Bristol once said: 'Your patients won't care how much you know, but they will know how much you care.' He was talking about caring for animals but he might just as well have been talking about people. Part of caring for people as a doctor is behaving in a way which is both ethically and legally acceptable. You could be the most knowl-edgeable doctor in the world, or the most technically competent in a given clinical area, but without an ethical base to your medical practice, how good a doctor will you really be?

It wasn't all that long ago that the sum total of teaching for the average British medical graduate consisted of a one-hour lecture by the dean in which the students were exhorted:

■ not to advertise their services
■ not to get drunk on duty
■ not to seduce their married patients.

These were popularly known as the three As (**A**dvertising, **A**lcohol and **A**dultery). There was little, if any, opportunity for students to engage in formal discussion of ethical problems in medicine. Rather, it was assumed that the new medical graduate would be able to cope, surrounded as he or she was by what Professor Len Doyal has described as 'well-disposed physicians'. Of course these discussions still occurred informally, on or off the ward, in the bar, in the mess and in the library, but often without any authoritative teaching to assist the students or young doctors in dealing with their inevitable concerns.

We firmly believe that most people who choose to study and practise medicine do so with the best of intentions and motivations. They want to be – and be recognised by others as – good doctors. We asked a group of junior doctors how they defined the qualities of a 'good' doctor. They defined these as being:

- a good communicator
- clinically competent and aware of their own limitations
- an improver of other people's health and facilitator of access to healthcare
- a teacher – of patients, families, other doctors and medical students, other health professionals and themselves too as a lifelong learner
- good listener and able to explain clearly
- empathetic and sympathetic
- patient and tolerant; non-discriminatory
- genuine and kind
- non-judgemental
- fair and trustworthy.

The list is not comprehensive or exclusive, nor does it mean that you will display all of these qualities on any one given day. Contrary to the unreasonable expectations of some, doctors and medical students are human beings too, and so they are fallible, imperfect, and likely to under-perform or even fail on occasions. Sometimes the pressures of working in medicine and in the health service can affect one's ability to be as good a doctor as one would want to be or should be. Patients can be amazingly forgiving and tolerant when doctors make mistakes, *if* that doctor displays some humility, says sorry when appropriate, appears caring and keeps the patient informed of what is happening.

However, the above list *is* aspirational. It shows that, despite all the pressures and the all-too-frequent criticism of the medical profession, the majority of doctors regard what they do as more than just a job, and – now and then – recognise what a huge privilege it is to be part of one of the most respected professions. Most doctors are conscientious individuals who reflect on the way they practise, occasionally to the point of obsession – they are concerned about getting it right.

Ethics (like the practice of medicine) is rarely about black and white, it is about learning to discern the shades of grey, dealing with uncertainty and finding the best possible course of action under the circumstances. We hope that this book will help you to think through possible courses of action or inaction in relation to the cases we have presented, the majority of which are drawn from personal experience and real life. This book is intended to help doctors and students preparing for college and medical school examinations, as well as helping those preparing for the ethical components of the General Medical Council's (GMC's) PLAB test; students may find it useful for coursework. We hope it will also help to reduce some of the anxiety when you are faced with an ethical dilemma at 3 am.

Although the book is aimed primarily at readers based in the UK, we hope that the range of cases presented from around the world will make it useful to a wider audience. However, we should point out that, throughout the text, references will be made to the UK legal systems, the GMC and the National Health Service (NHS). Readers in other jurisdictions will need to clarify the prevailing law and ethical guidelines pertaining to their location.

We thank the readers of the first edition for their continued support and welcome any comments which could help us further improve the content of this book for future editions.

Chapter Two

HOW TO STUDY ETHICS AND LAW

The first thing to say about studying medical ethics and law is: start with an open mind.

Medical students and doctors should know about relevant ethico-legal aspects of their profession at all levels of their careers. A formal assessment of the knowledge of ethics and law is becoming increasingly important as the government and GMC are requiring doctors and medical students to know what is expected of them; ignorance is not a defence. Medical schools and Royal Colleges are therefore examining ethics and law more overtly and more thoroughly.

You will also be assessed on ethico-legal issues in job interviews. You may be presented with a scenario or vignette similar to the ones described in the OSCE section below. Not only is ethical competence increasingly a requirement for most jobs, but it is also an excellent way of finding out what you are like as a person and a colleague – so be prepared!

HOW TO REVISE AND PASS THE EXAMS

What are OSCEs and what do they do?

Objective Structured Clinical Examinations (OSCEs) are now being used widely to examine students and doctors. They are primarily used to help assess clinical and communication skills as well as professional behaviour and attitudes; they are also used to assess knowledge about ethical and legal issues.

OSCE formats

The format for these examinations varies. An OSCE is usually made up of several 'stations', with each station lasting between five and ten minutes. A station is often a structured viva with certain props such as X-rays, blood results and anatomical models. Real or standardised patients are frequently used too, especially to assess communication and examination skills. At least one examiner is there to watch how you perform, ask you questions, or play a specific role, eg as a patient.

Marking

Marking schemes also vary. Examiners will assess you by using a checklist of items or a global rating scale or a mixture of both.

- **Checklists** mean that you will only get credit for doing the things on the checklist. Your final mark for the station will be a reflection of how

9

many items you managed to do successfully. However, checklists do not let you get more marks for doing extra things not included on the checklist.

- **Global rating scales** mean that the examiner will look at your performance as a whole and give you the mark that is most appropriate. A marking guide is often followed so that the examiner is aware of what standard of performance equates to which mark.

The global rating scales allow examiners to give credit to a student who achieves everything required in a courteous, confident manner, whereas a checklist may dictate that such a candidate receives the same mark as a student who does everything in a hesitant and disrespectful way. Most examining bodies employ a mixture of both assessment formats. Examiners use a checklist to help them assess performance but ultimately they are asked to write down the mark they feel most appropriate, based on overall competence.

Passing

Generally speaking, in order to do very well in an OSCE you will have to do well in most stations. To fail you have to perform poorly in most stations – most people pass. There are three main ways in which examining bodies decide who passes and who fails:

- **Criterion-referenced grading** means that candidates are assessed against a set of criteria and must achieve a minimum standard or percentage (the 'pass mark') to pass. This percentage is usually set before the exam takes place. Criterion-referencing means that as long as you achieve the predetermined percentage you will pass, no matter how many other candidates achieve the standard. However, if the exam is harder or easier than usual, it becomes unfair as fewer or more students, respectively, will manage to pass.
- **Norm-referenced grading** means that students are judged against each other. After the exam, all the marks are placed on a graph. A normal distribution curve (a bell-shaped line) inevitably results, due to the fact that a small number of students do very well and a small number do poorly, with the majority achieving somewhere in-between. Statistical analyses of these results allow examining bodies to set a pass mark based on the performance of the students, so that the standard of the exam itself is less important. Norm-referencing is sometimes preferred because it is difficult to ensure that exactly the same standard of exam can be reproduced year after year. It is also good because you are compared against your peers, not against an arbitrary percentage. However, it also means that some students will

inevitably fail each time, independent of their final percentage. The Royal Colleges typically use this type of grading to decide which candidates pass and fail their Membership exams.

■ **Pass/fail criteria.** Some stations have a pass/fail criterion which means that if you fail to do something then you will automatically fail the station no matter how well you perform overall. The pass/fail criterion is often something either very basic or very important, and usually it is both, eg failing to check that other people are standing clear of the patient before shocking during advanced life support. It is also possible that an OSCE will have a pass/fail *station* which means that if you fail that station you will automatically fail the entire OSCE – no matter what your total score. Again, this station is likely to be examining something like basic life support – a fundamental skill. Most medical schools do not use pass/fail criteria and do not have pass/fail stations.

Ethics and law in OSCEs

There are several ways in which ethics and law can be brought into OSCEs.

A *whole* station may be purely about ethico-legal issues, as in the MRCP Part 2 PACES and PLAB exams. You will be required to discuss ethico-legal issues for five to ten minutes with an examiner or do a role-play in that time. Real-life examples that the authors have encountered are:

■ Good medical practice – Talking about what you would do if one of your colleagues was on drugs/alcohol and potentially unsafe to practise.

■ Treatment in the best interests of the patient – How to deal with an unconscious patient who has attempted suicide.

■ Explaining to a patient whose conduct presents a risk to others (eg the epileptic patient who drives) that confidentiality is not absolute.

■ Mental Health Act – When and why it may be necessary to section someone and how you should go about it.

■ Criteria for informed consent of treatment, eg talking to a parent about an investigation or procedure for their child.

■ Assessing Fraser competence – Deciding whether an adolescent has sufficient understanding to make their own healthcare decisions.

■ Assessment of capacity – Deciding whether a confused patient is able to consent to an investigation or procedure.

■ Refusal of consent to an operation – How to deal with this ethically and legally when the patient is competent.

- Breaching confidentiality – What to do if you suspect child abuse/bullying.
- Explaining to a senior colleague about working on a research team that uses animal subjects.
- Assessing your honesty and willingness to 'bluff' by asking you to explain something rare or specialised (and of which you are not expected to have heard) to a colleague.

Ethico-legal issues can also form *part* of a station. You may be required to draw upon and demonstrate ethico-legal knowledge in stations primarily designed to test other skills or knowledge. This happens in many different scenarios and we have come across it in stations concerning:

- taking a history of child abuse
- discussion of a positive result for a sexually transmitted infection with a patient
- doing a cervical smear and colposcopy exam
- discussion of breastfeeding with a new mother – respecting her right to choose, even if it is not in her child's best medical interests
- management of a patient who has taken a paracetamol overdose
- doing any kind of clinical exam, eg thyroid, rectal, chest – obtaining consent
- suspected tuberculosis infection – how to deal with a notifiable disease.

Your situation

In order to prepare for an OSCE it is helpful to think about your own situation.

- What kind of skills, knowledge and behaviour is usually examined?
- What stations have been used in the past?
- What are the obvious ethico-legal areas that can be examined as entire stations?
- Are there any other stations that might involve ethico-legal aspects while primarily assessing other skills/knowledge?

Ten top tips for OSCEs

Before the OSCE

1 Practise the skills in preparation for the OSCE.

Practice (with feedback) is the best way to improve any skill. In terms of ethico-legal skills, this means confronting yourself with ethical and legal problems and thinking about how you would deal with them. The cases in this book will help you prepare, but you should also use your own experience on the wards to help you develop your thoughts and skills. Work in groups so that you can give feedback to each other. Use the questions on the previous page to tailor your revision to your own situation.

2 Get a good night's sleep before the exam.

OSCEs are usually about how you perform skills and not about reproducing isolated facts. While you may feel that it is sometimes better to stay up late revising for an MCQ exam (multiple choice question exam, which purely tests knowledge), an OSCE is a test that requires you to be fully mentally alert. You will not make a good impression if you look tired, unshaven or are scruffily dressed. Be well rested and confident.

During the OSCE

3 Be prepared for ethico-legal issues to come up.

Do not be blinkered into seeing only clinical knowledge and skills as being relevant. Be aware that, just as in everyday clinical practice, ethics and law pervades most aspects of medical care and therefore may come up in nearly any OSCE station.

4 Cite the issues that make the problem ethically or legally difficult.

When faced with an ethical dilemma such as the poorly performing colleague who may be endangering patient care, take a while to think about the issues before opening your mouth. For example, the fact that the colleague is a doctor and has a duty to their patients, the fact that you are a doctor (or medical student) and have a similar duty to patients, and that 'telling on' your colleague may not necessarily achieve the best outcome. Take your time to think about the problem from all angles. Show the examiner that you are exploring all the issues without rushing into action. Doing this will also give you time to think.

5 Take your time to go through the steps in your thought process.

Do not come up with solutions straight away. Examiners want to see that you are a careful decision-maker and that you will take time to examine the issues before making a judgement. They want you to demonstrate that you will think through such difficult problems in a clear and stepwise fashion. This shows that you are not simply a robot who has learned the 'answers' to several different ethical dilemmas, but that you are a thinking person who will address each situation on a case-by-case basis.

6 Know about the GMC's 'duties of a doctor' guidance.

These handbooks should be read before the exam so you can refer to them during the OSCE. You don't have to know page numbers or anything, but you should at least be aware that they exist and that they provide guidance on your responsibilities as a doctor. Mention them in the exam if it is relevant to do so.

7 Back up your thoughts by referring to ethical principles and approaches; show awareness of legal terms.

Refer by name to any ethical principles that you use, eg beneficence, utilitarianism. Explain any legal background to terms such as 'negligence' or 'capacity to give informed consent' if relevant – though this tip will earn you brownie points only if you know what you are talking about! Do not use words if you are not sure what they mean because examiners will pick up on this and quiz you until you feel as if you do not know anything at all. Stick to what you know, but if you know any ethical principles or legal terms, so much the better.

8 Seek help.

The complicated nature of ethico-legal problems means that you would be unwise to act alone. Always say that you would seek help from a suitable source, such as a defence organisation or a senior. Bear in mind the importance of safeguarding confidentiality when saying that you would do this.

9 Start each station with a positive attitude.

If you feel that you have done badly in a station, forget about it as soon as the bell goes. Put it out of your mind and go into the next station with a clear head, fresh start and confident approach. Remember that to do badly in an OSCE you would have to do poorly in *most* stations. Even candidates who gain top marks tend to have at least one station that did not go well.

After the OSCE

10 Relax with your mates.

The OSCE is often a very stressful experience because it usually requires you to demonstrate a diverse range of skills under time pressure. It is important to relax and unwind afterwards in whichever way you please. Dissect the exam with your friends if you must, but remember that the OSCE is a very individual experience and it is almost impossible to know how your performance compares with anyone else's. Wait until the results come out before you cancel your summer holiday!

Ethics and law in essays

Most of us will not have had much practice at essay writing, especially now that medical schools are moving away from using essays to assess knowledge. Despite this, it is still a useful skill to learn and will help you in the future when you are asked to write papers, reports and book chapters.

Essay formats and marking

Writing essays in ethics and law can come in various formats – they can be as a Special Study Module (SSM) or Student Selected Component (SSC), a piece of coursework, or a formal exam under the pressure of time.

Essays can be marked in various ways. Sometimes examiners will use a checklist to ensure that you have covered the relevant points. You may also get credit for writing well; a clear structure and style, logical arguments and conclusions, spelling and referencing are all important.

Ten top tips for writing an essay

Before the essay

1   Have a positive attitude.

OK, so you may not rate yourself as much of a writer but doing an essay is not that scary. You are intelligent, can think logically and can cope with new challenges – that is all you need to start off with. You can do this.

2   Pick a topic that interests you and formulate a hypothesis.

Whether it is for a piece of coursework or an exam, you will often be given several options from which to choose a topic to write about. Think about issues that grab you and stimulate you in some way. It need not be something you know a lot about already, but if the topic inspires you to *think* in the first place, then you will learn much more easily. For long essays or a dissertation it is helpful if you can choose a subject which you have personal experience of, one which is topical or one where you have access to original sources; it will keep you interested and will make your work original. In the early stages it is much better to be passionate about the subject than to know a lot about it.

Your hypothesis can be tentative at first but should address a specific issue. Anything else you write in the essay can only really be justified in terms of how it relates back to this thesis. If your question is set, you must make sure you answer it.

3 Increase your background knowledge of the subject; discuss your thoughts with others.

Research the topic in the library and use secondary sources to gain access to primary sources, but try to read the primary sources. Use journals (eg the *Journal of Medical Ethics* or the *Medical Law Review*), as well as books, so that you learn about how different people have approached the topic, particularly recently. Compare your viewpoint with theirs: Do they agree with you? In what respect do they disagree with you? What are the flaws in their arguments? All this can be included in your essay.

Debating the issues with others will help you to detect holes in your arguments, and develop a wider perspective. The good thing about this is that you can start up discussions with anyone who's interested. Most people have opinions even if they can't back them up very well. Talk to other students, doctors, patients, or your family and friends – this is what happens in real practice.

Good note taking is an investment in your essay that you will never regret. Be sure to note the source of any information (and especially quotations) so that you can find it later. Make reference to all relevant information as you go along. This will also avoid inadvertent plagiarism and incomplete referencing which is very important in a subject such as ethics which relies on some level of original thought. Use of a computer to cut and paste notes will save you time and will avoid mistakes in duplications.

4 Reassess your hypothesis.

At this stage, you will be able to reassess your focus in the light of all your new information. Formulate your thesis definitively and break it into the main issues that you need to cover to make you argument logical. If you use a spider diagram to note down your ideas and the main aspects that you are going to address, then it will be easy for you to spot links between issues and arguments.

5 Make a plan.

This is the key to a good essay. If you have a good plan, then your writing will flow much better. Formulate your spider diagram into a plan that looks something along the lines of:

■ introduction – the context of the problem or case description
■ breakdown of the relevant ethical and legal issues, definition of terms
■ examination of each issue in turn – what your argument is, the opposing position and why your position is stronger
■ summary of the final conclusion.

Your plan should be more detailed than this, and you should be able to use the sub-headings in your final essay. If possible, discuss your plan with your supervisor so that they can give you some feedback on your ideas and so that you can make sure you are on the right track. In an exam, make sure you put a line through your plan before handing it in.

During the essay

6 Be disciplined and start writing.

You'll need to get yourself into a quiet place with no distractions. Most people prefer to write on a computer but you must do what you are most comfortable with. If you prefer to handwrite your work, then get lots of paper and a good pen. The hardest thing about writing an essay is getting started. Do not make it into a psychological barrier that you have to break through. Just sit down and do it. You can always change the introduction later on if you are not happy with it. If necessary, you can create rewards for yourself when you have achieved certain targets along the way. Chocolate is always a good one, but it could be anything that you enjoy. Make sure you take regular breaks too – most people find it difficult to concentrate after 30 minutes or so, but don't stop if you are in full flow.

7 Style points.

■ Guide the reader through your essay using sub-headings and signposting words (eg when listing different points use first, second, third, etc).
■ Try to structure each section according to the same principles in a kind of iterative process:
   ▪ Present an idea
   ↓
   ▪ Write a supporting statement
   ▪ Elaborate on the supporting statement
   ↓
   ▪ Write another supporting statement
   ▪ Elaborate on this supporting statement ⌐┘
   ↓
   ▪ Conclude/summarise the section.

- Give illustrations and definitions and use elaborations on arguments, cross-referencing and repetition back to your hypothesis.
- Use quotations carefully. Instead of quoting whole paragraphs, make quotations concise and relevant to support your thesis.

8   Don't worry about:

- the word count – you will find enough to write about; just make sure you do not waffle or repeat yourself; if you exceed the word limit, editing can be left until the end. Be sure to seek guidance on how flexible the word limit is.
- getting stuck – take a break, go and do something else, talk to your supervisor.
- using simple language – write in the best way you can to express what you think. It is always better to say complicated things in a simple way than simple things in a complicated way. Keep sentences short, rather than too long.

9   Check through the essay before handing it in.

Get other people to read it through too if possible, to get a fresh perspective on what you have written. Sometimes you can get so close to it that you fail to see obvious mistakes. If you have time, leave the essay alone for a few days and look at it again yourself. It should be easy to read, flow logically, be well structured with headings and have each argument backed up with references. Don't forget to check your spelling!

After the essay

10 Get feedback.

You may want to forget about the essay once you have handed it in. However, use each assignment as an opportunity to get better. Try to get specific feedback from the examiner about areas you can improve for next time. Examples of common problems include lack of clarity in your explanation, illogical steps in your arguments, or being too waffly.

Good sources for help include the website www.write-an-essay.com, and *The Oxford Guide to Writing* by Thomas Kane (Oxford University Press, 1983). If you are having a specific problem with your essay, speak to your course instructor.

TAKING MEDICAL ETHICS AND LAW FURTHER

If you are thinking about studying medical ethics and law in greater depth there are several options open to you. You could decide to do an SSM or SCC, an intercalated Bachelor of Science (BSc) or even a postgraduate degree. There are many reasons why you might like to spend time studying medical ethics and law. The following are just a few.

Interest in the subject; desire to take a year out of science

The main reason should be that you are interested the subject. In fact, it would be very difficult to maintain your motivation in *any* discipline unless you are interested in it. As a medical student or doctor you might have spent most of your time in formal education increasing your knowledge of science and developing a scientific approach to problems. This is undoubtedly useful but there is a lot more to medicine than science. Studying philosophy, ethics and law can help you to think 'outside the box' and appreciate different aspects of human problems.

Wish to develop your own ethical beliefs and debating skills

Most people can say *what* they think or believe about a particular ethical dilemma but often find it difficult to say *why* they think a certain way and therefore fail to convince others. Good philosophers and lawyers can argue their case and defend their points with well-reasoned thoughts and evidence. You may be keen to develop your own debating skills and wish to learn how to structure your arguments to justify your position – studying ethics and law will give you the knowledge and the tools to do this more convincingly.

Wish to improve your essay-writing technique

The ability to write essays is a useful skill and can help to improve your written communication. However, it is not an easy technique to learn and is often avoided by most people. Medical ethics and law courses usually involve a lot of essay writing. It can be very difficult at first but lecturers are used to dealing with students who have little experience of essay writing and will often give very good support.

19

Wish to enhance your clinical practice

Once you are working, you may not feel confident about your level of knowledge of medical ethics and law, and you may feel that you find it difficult to know what is the 'right' thing to do in certain situations. Even medical students and junior doctors can find themselves in ethical and legal dilemmas, and not knowing what to do can lead to potentially serious consequences. Defence organisations can offer advice but sometimes this is difficult or impossible to obtain. The more senior and experienced you become, the more responsibility you will have and the more important and difficult the decisions you will be required to make. Learning about ethics and law will give you the opportunity to gain knowledge and skills that will help you to enhance your clinical practice.

Getting an extra qualification

An intercalated degree is definitely a good bargain – you get the equivalent of a three-year degree for the price of one. If you want to do a BSc because you would like some extra letters after your name, that is fair enough since it will be an advantage to your career. However, it is important to pick a subject you enjoy. Spending a year forcing yourself to become immersed in something you dislike is a recipe for torture and failure. If you cannot find anything you like at the moment, then wait a year or two. There are always new courses starting up on different subjects in different places. Most medical schools allow you to intercalate at any time before your final year. Further possibilities will be open to you as you continue in your postgraduate career, eg a master's or PhD degree. Medical ethics and law is also available as an MA or MSc, so you could always pursue the interest after you have graduated from medicine instead of doing an intercalated BSc.

Spending an extra year as a student

This may be seen as a disadvantage by some people but it can also be a plus point. There are, of course, some problems: you may drop a year behind friends who continue on the clinical track, your debt will increase, you may feel that you will forget some medical knowledge and skills during your year 'out'. Most people experience these problems, but to a much smaller degree than they expected:

- Instead of losing friends, you gain them. It is usually easy to keep up with friends from your former year group while making new ones in your new year group. It can also be useful to have good mates in the year above who can tell you what to expect in exams and teach you on the wards.
- Money can be a worry and if it is an issue for you, there are trust funds around which may be able to help. Speak to your medical society, faculty, students union and bank about ways in which you can minimise the financial burden of extending your studies. If you are pursuing a postgraduate degree, look out for scholarships and bursaries, as well as locum work.
- Forgetting medical knowledge happens to some extent but you will be surprised by how much you retain. You will also be at an advantage compared with others as you will know a lot of ethics and law which will be useful for your medical exams at both undergraduate and postgraduate levels.

Being a student is ultimately very enjoyable and allows you to take some more long summer holidays – which you will miss greatly once you start work. Make the most of it!

PICKING A COURSE

Many universities offer courses in medical ethics and law, and you do not have to go to your local institution, so it is worth investigating the alternatives. There are some factors which you may want to take into account.

Method of teaching

Discussions and debates based on relevant problems are the best and usually the most enjoyable way in which to learn medical ethics and law. If the intercalated BSc is run jointly with a postgraduate course, then you will have joint classes with people who are healthcare professionals themselves as well as students. This can make for very lively and interesting discussions as many people will have real-life experience which can be brought into group sessions. This can also be very motivating and allows you to learn a great deal more about practical applications of ethico-legal principles.

Flexibility of the course to suit your interests

Is the course modular? Which parts are compulsory and what are the options available to choose from?

Method of assessment

Will you be assessed continuously or by an exam at the end? There may be a mixture of both. It is likely that most courses will use essay assignments to evaluate students but there may be other methods used, such as MCQs or oral presentations. Choose an assessment style that suits the way you work.

Students' and teachers' views

Speak to people who are on the course or who have completed it; arrange a meeting with one of the lecturers or course organisers.

What are the students' views? Did they enjoy the course? If they had difficulties, was there good support from the lecturers? Do the course organisers listen to suggestions on ways to improve the course and has action been taken in response to problems? Good and enthusiastic lecturers will be only too pleased to discuss the course with you.

Location

It is a good idea to familiarise yourself with the location and investigate areas such as accommodation, the student union, facilities, libraries, etc. Moving away for a year can be difficult initially but often allows for a richer experience.

If you are doing the course by distance learning, you should make sure there are opportunities for regular contact with other students on your course as well as the teachers. Distance learning requires more motivation than classroom-based courses but may suit people who are unable to move to the location of the course.

Chapter Three

HOW TO TEACH MEDICAL ETHICS AND LAW

'Doctor' literally means 'teacher', and we recognise that doctors and medical students teach one another from a very early stage of training. One of the most important areas of medicine you might find yourself teaching is about how to be an ethical doctor and how to practise ethical medicine. In this chapter we aim to provide some practical advice on how to teach the ethics of medicine and the ethical values of the medical profession.

TEACHING ETHICS AND LAW IN PRACTICE

You do not have to be trained in educational techniques to be an effective teacher for others. Doctors do most of their teaching in an informal way in the clinical setting, with learners observing as well as being actively instructed. There are several concepts to bear in mind when teaching ethics and law in this situation. They can be summarised in the mnemonic **ETHICS**.

Example

Leading by example is a very powerful method that you can use to teach others. If you model ethical behaviour in your clinical practice, you will have a profound effect on the way others think and behave. It does not matter how often students are told to act in a certain way, if they do not see their seniors doing it themselves, they will not do it. Training to be a doctor is like an apprenticeship, and you will be a role model for your juniors, whether you are aware of it or not.

Talk

Actually discussing ethical issues is a very effective way of allowing learners to examine their own values and compare them with others' values. Getting learners to verbalise their thoughts and decision-making processes prompts them to scrutinise their attitudes and forces them to justify what they believe. You may find that you will learn as much as they will from these types of discussion.

Help

Helping students to come to conclusions is part of the role you will play as their teacher. Ethics is not a 'right or wrong' discipline where answers can be memorised. You, as their senior, should not aim to impose your own beliefs on your students. Instead, work with them in the search for what each of you considers to be an acceptable moral solution.

Inspire

If you can inspire your students to take an interest in the subject you wish them to learn, you will be more than halfway there. Find out what interests them and tailor your teaching to what they want to learn, rather than what you think they should know. If students are encouraged and motivated they will learn more effectively than if they are simply lectured at. You can still teach them what you think is relevant, but try to relate it to something that they find important.

Context

Always set the subject in context, rather than referring to abstract problems. As illustrated by the cases in this book, ethics and law pervades many aspects of medical care, and you will not have to look very hard to find ethico-legal dilemmas in everyday situations. Use examples of real cases that the students see on the wards or in clinics to start a discussion on ethics. By doing this, students are more likely to remember the concepts clearly because they will also remember the patient involved. This will also encourage them to see the relevance of what they are learning.

Stimulate

Asking stimulating questions can have several purposes: it will encourage students to examine their own knowledge and attitudes; it can help to enthuse students and arouse their curiosity in the issues; it will allow you to get an idea of how much your students already know about a topic. By challenging them in this way, they will also learn more effectively and will develop a deeper appreciation of the subject. Questioning is most effective in promoting learning when it is done in a supportive atmosphere, rather than with the aim of embarrassing or exposing students' lack of knowledge. Working together with your students in a collaborative way can help to foster a good learning environment and is more productive than being confrontational.

SOME FREQUENTLY ASKED QUESTIONS ABOUT TEACHING MEDICAL ETHICS AND LAW

Don't you need a qualification to teach medical ethics and law?

No – medical ethics is frequently taught in an informal way (eg during a grand round presentation, or in a general practitioner's (GP's) surgery after a patient has left the room, or in a discussion following a hospital ward round) by clinicians at all levels and by those with an interest in the subject. However, there are also many taught or research courses available that do lead to a formal qualification in medical ethics and law, ranging from a certificate up to PhD level. Contact your local university or library to check on the availability of courses in your area. Doctors, dentists and other health professionals in training may find that there is a generic skills programme available in their region or specialty that includes a medical ethics module. Most medical schools in the UK now include formal and structured teaching in medical ethics and law throughout their undergraduate curriculum, and opportunities often exist to become involved in this teaching.

So how can I teach medical ethics and law myself?

Make use of cases you have encountered, experienced or read about. Every doctor and health professional develops a repertoire or repository of stories; many of these have educational value. Medicine is very much an oral culture which benefits from the telling of stories – how often have you heard a doctor or other health professional start a medical conversation by saying, 'I had this case once' or, 'I knew a patient who . . .'? This can often help others learn about how to deal with a current dilemma.

The phrases 'corridor medicine' or 'car park medicine' illustrate the way in which practical ethics is frequently taught and learnt on the hoof as it were – when doctors and health professionals meet one another in passing, and exchange questions, ideas and information. Be careful to reflect on the need to respect patient confidentiality, and be cautious of telling stories that reflect badly on a colleague without their consent.

Any tips for making ethics and law teaching relevant and interesting?

- Encourage discussion of ethical issues; relate them to cases observed in primary care surgeries or home visits, out-patient clinics, ward rounds and in theatre.

- Invite learners to share their experiences of ethical dilemmas.
- Set up a debate on a current ethical dilemma in the public domain.
- Use references to the media (newspapers, news programmes and magazines often cover ethical issues in some depth) and popular culture – the American television series *ER* is a fantastic source of ethical triggers, as are the British *Casualty* and other medically related series.

How can I keep up to date on ethico-legal cases?

- Read the journals – the *Journal of Medical Ethics*, the *BMJ*, the *Lancet*, the *New England Journal of Medicine*, the *American Journal of Bioethics*; all these (and many others) publish a wide variety of ethics cases and developments.
- Use the media – newspapers, news programmes and the Internet provide a wealth of resources. The appendix at the end of this book has a list of web-based and other resources, which may prove helpful.

DESIGNING AN ETHICS COURSE

The team that has written this book includes several medical teachers who have run ethics and law courses over a number of years in medical schools and universities around the world. Many of the lessons we have learnt from our experiences may be relevant to others developing an ethics course at any level – undergraduate, postgraduate or continuing education.

- **Keep it real** – Apply theory to practice wherever possible, so that relevance and utility are both clear.
- **Cover a range of topics** – Don't just concentrate on your own research interests.
- **Identify learners' needs** – In simple terms, ask your students what they think they know and (where possible) try to address these needs.
- **Make it lively** – Use quizzes, buzz groups, student-led debates and discussions, small-group and plenary presentations.
- Develop a **student and patient-centred approach**, where shared values, personal experiences and individual opinions are prized and promoted.
- Take a **case-based** approach to the teaching – Enable and facilitate discussion of cases that are both authentic and present an ethical challenge.

- **Employ humanistic values** – Treat the students with respect and kindness as this helps to develop their own sense of collegiality. Engage with all participants, not just the confident and vocal students.
- **Create the right atmosphere** – Encourage an interactive, non-dogmatic, supportive climate in both plenary sessions and small-group work, eg use students' names and assign roles, such as student chairs (who run the session), scribes (who write a summary of the discussions on a flip chart) and rapporteurs (who report and represent the views of the group's members).
- **Create a safe environment** – Let students (and teachers) be unafraid to voice their own opinions and be able to tolerate, understand and even accept views and perspectives different from their own.
- **Recruit faculty with care** – Ensure that those who teach ethics and facilitate discussions have the appropriate skills and sensitivity; for facilitators, in-depth training in ethics is less important than being open-minded, and having the ability to get on with learners, listening to them and being honest with them.
- **Venues matter** – Choose venues which are appropriate to the type of teaching and learning chosen for the course, eg a lecture theatre for plenary presentations and discussion, smaller rooms for small-group work.
- **Don't forget the administration** – Ensure that room and equipment bookings are made in good time, that a timetable and programme are sent well in advance to both faculty and students, and that handouts, evaluation sheets and other materials are prepared in good time for the course.
- **Structure the programme** – Organisation and preparation of teaching and learning help to promote a sense of confidence and security in both students and teachers; this includes provision of a detailed timetable, while allowing for expressed learning needs to be met.

Chapter Four

THE BASICS OF MEDICAL ETHICS AND LAW

PHILOSOPHICAL

We have produced a 'rough guide' to help you understand the philosophical jargon, as well as the origins of and ideas behind the main ethical theories. This glossary will be useful for examinations, for writing essays and for when you are reading ethical texts.

Ethics and morality

The terms 'ethics' (ethical) and 'morality' (moral) can have different meanings. Some people see '**morality**' as referring to an individual's or a group's sense of right and wrong and '**ethics**' as concerning the critical scrutiny of such moral beliefs, looking at (for example) how logical or coherent the beliefs are. Others, however, have used the terms interchangeably. Whichever view is preferred, ethics/morality is all about right, wrong, good, bad – in short, it is concerned with the 'ought' rather than the 'is'.

In the following sections we start at an abstract level, outlining some of the main theories of ethics that have relevance to healthcare. We then move closer to practice, describing the popular 'four principles' approach to healthcare ethics. We conclude with some examples of codes of ethics, which build on the theories and relate even more directly to practice, since they provide healthcare professionals with a chance to profess the ethical commitments of their profession(s).

Utilitarianism/consequentialism

One of the central questions of ethics is, 'What should I do?'. Consequentialists think you should do that which has the best consequences. Utilitarianism is a prominent type of consequentialist thought and is largely attributed to the work of Jeremy Bentham and John Stuart Mill in the nineteenth century. Utilitarianism argues that the correct action is that which gives the 'greatest good for the greatest number'. This requires calculation of outcomes and of the predicted benefit that these will provide for both individuals and society. For example, utilitarians might argue that it would be acceptable to kill one person in order to save the lives of 1000 people. You may also encounter the distinction between 'act' and 'rule' utilitarianism. Briefly, this describes whether one looks to the *act per se* to assess the moral value of a decision or to the moral value of the *rule that would be created* by carrying out a particular act.

Kantianism/deontology

Deontologists think the answer to the question, 'What should I do?' is that you should do that which it is your duty to do. Immanuel Kant, an eighteenth century Prussian philosopher, is considered to be the founding father of deontological thinking. He said that some things are just 'right' – he defines all kinds of 'right' and 'wrong' without reference to the consequences that might follow from a rule. Kant explains rules in which he states man *ought* or *ought not* to behave in a particular way (duties) as the 'categorical imperative'. He stated that you should never treat people as a means to an end, but always as an 'end in themselves'. In other words, you should never subject a human being to anything that is not 'right', even if the result is that many more people will benefit, eg killing one person in order to save 1000 people would be unacceptable because it would mean that one person is subjected to an act that is wrong.

Rights

According to some people, rights are the flip side of duties. In order to have a right, there is a corresponding duty on others to ensure that this right is not infringed. This means that, for example, you are not allowed to kill someone because this would impinge on their right to life. Some matters are considered to be basic human rights, and these have even gained legal protection (see legal section below).

Virtue ethics

Virtue ethicists think the deontologists and utilitarians are asking the wrong question – for them, the important question is, 'Who should I be?' (or 'How should I live?'). They think it is most important to be a virtuous person, where a virtue is a mean between two excesses. For example, courage is a virtue (good character trait) because it strikes the right balance between cowardliness and foolhardiness. Although it may be harder to translate into rules or codes of conduct, this approach is still important in medical practice and training, because you will undoubtedly learn from the example set by your teachers and colleagues. (Are they 'good' or 'bad' doctors?)

Feminist ethics

Feminists criticise those social institutions and structures that work for the benefit of men and disbenefit of women. Feminist ethicists look to understand gender relationships and remove bias towards men. They stress the role and importance of an 'ethics of care' which emphasises emotion and interpersonal relationships over 'objective' reason and logic.

Narrative ethics

Narrative ethics takes people's lives in their individual context into account when determining what is ethically correct or incorrect. It dismisses rules and principles as having inherent value per se, requiring instead that all moral decision-making takes place in context. The aim is not generalisability but rich understanding of individual circumstances.

The four principles of bioethics

Many of you will be introduced to medical ethics at your medical school through the 'four principles' framework. The four principles are:

- **Respect for autonomy** – The principle of 'self-rule'. People should be allowed to make their own decisions about what happens to them.
- **Beneficence** – Do good.
- **Non-maleficence** – This comes from the Latin phrase *primum non nocere*, which means 'above all, do no harm'.
- **Justice** – Ensuring that people are treated fairly and equally.

These principles, coined by Tom Beauchamp and James Childress, two American philosophers, can be used as a tool for structuring your thoughts when you are first faced with ethical dilemmas. They enable you to give initial consideration as to how best to deal with problems. However, many other theories explore further aspects of philosophy. By using the four principles in combination with some of these other ideas, you will be able to give a more complete argument and therefore address ethical problems more effectively. Furthermore, you may want to break down some of the principles when using the model. For example, when considering autonomy, you could also ask how one can maximise or impede autonomy as a doctor; and or when considering justice, you could refer to other theorists such as John Rawls or Robert Nozick to explain how you are interpreting and applying the concept of justice.

Paternalism/parentalism

One way of understanding the doctor–patient relationship is a scenario in which the doctor is the 'expert' and determines what is best for the patient. The doctor acts as the patient's 'parent' and tells them what to do, even making choices on their behalf (eg withholding information on the grounds that it is too complex or distressing for a patient). Fortunately, this behaviour is less common nowadays, and has been replaced to a greater or lesser degree by respect for patient autonomy. Indeed, the GMC explicitly states that a competent patient's best interests can only be understood meaningfully by reference to what the patient him- or herself believes and wishes.

Codes of ethics

Hippocratic Oath

The Hippocratic Oath was the first known ethical code of conduct for doctors. It was composed by the 'Father of Medicine', Hippocrates (born circa 406 BC on the Greek island of Kos). The Oath encouraged the teaching medicine, acting in the best interests of patients and abstaining from whatever is deleterious and mischievous, and maintaining patient confidentiality. However, it also outlawed abortion and gave emphasis to principles such as paternalism. The original Oath is no longer taken in most medical schools.

Many people (including medical students and doctors) still believe that the Hippocratic Oath is sworn by, and binding upon, doctors, but it rarely, if ever, is in modern medical practice. However, it remains interesting as an example of the long history of professional codes of conduct in medicine and as a starting point for mapping the evolution of medical ethics and professional self-regulation.

Helsinki Declaration and Geneva Declaration

More recent codes were developed in response to the atrocities of the two world wars and came about as a result of the Nuremburg War Trials where Nazi doctors were found guilty of conducting experiments on a range of people including Jews, homosexuals and disabled people. The declarations made recommendations covering both medical practice and research. Both declarations have been revised and updated since their first incarnations.

Medical school promises

Numerous medical schools worldwide have now developed their own promises based on the Hippocratic Oath and later declarations, which new doctors take on graduation. These are commonplace in America but less popular in the UK. They go by various names, but the most popular is probably the 'White Coat Ceremony'.

Why do you think that doctors, as a professional group, require professional codes of conduct and oaths? What is the moral rationale for these codes and ceremonies?

LEGAL

Ethics and law?

How, then, do ethics and the law interrelate? Some people might cynically claim that they do not but the truth is that they do, albeit not always in the most obvious ways. Legal philosophers, for example, study 'jurisprudence', which asks whether or not there is something intrinsically or necessarily 'moral' built into the very nature of 'law'. We do not need to examine this in any detail, as it is sufficient to note that the relationship between the two is also of real concern to healthcare professionals, patients and, indeed, lawmakers alike. Consider the following words of Lord Justice Ward, in an important recent judgment: 'It is . . . important to stress the obvious. This court is a court of law, not of morals, and our task has been to find, and our duty is then to apply, the relevant principles of law to the situation before us – a situation which is quite unique.'

The situation is not quite what Ward LJ claims, however. Certainly there are areas of the law which have little or nothing to do with ethics; equally, there are aspects of moral life that have not been (or cannot be) enshrined in law. But what Ward's statement overlooks is that much of UK medical law is in fact dependent to a large extent on ethical concepts.

Consider for a moment the situation that Ward himself was adjudicating. 'Jodie' and 'Mary' were conjoined twins, who were joined at the base of the spine. As Mary's heart and lungs did not function, she was dependent on her sister for her survival. The doctors felt that the strain would lead to the death of both twins within a matter of months. However, they felt that Jodie would have a good chance of (what the judges termed) a 'normal' life if she were to be separated from her dependent sister. Unfortunately, separation would mean the inevitable death of Mary. Many questions of law were involved. For criminal lawyers, the issue was: whether the doctors would be murdering Mary. For family lawyers the issue was: how the interests of both girls could be respected. Human rights lawyers, meanwhile, wondered how the balance could be struck between the equal right to life enjoyed by both sisters.

Notably, in resolving these issues and finding that surgical separation would be lawful, Ward LJ spent much of his judgment applying the principle of the sanctity of human life – an ethical principle. We do not need to stop there either. We saw in relation to the four principles how respect for patient autonomy has become increasingly important, and this ethical principle also finds great support in UK law. In a recent ruling in which the court confirmed that a paralysed woman had the right to refuse the artificial ventilation that was keeping her alive, one judge even made explicit reference to some of the philosophical literature about patient autonomy.

Ethics and law evidently do interrelate, especially in the area of healthcare. Of course, it will always be appropriate to debate and challenge the extent to which the law gets things (ethically) right.

The nature of law

That ethics and law are related should therefore be clear, but they also differ. Some of the scholars of jurisprudence claim that law is special because it is backed by sanctions; in other words, that law involves punishments or remedies (eg financial compensation). That is true but is it enough to define 'law'? You may instead think of law as a series of rules that exist to guide human activities. These rules can perform two general functions: they can proscribe (tell you what not to do) and prescribe (tell you what to do), and in prescribing they can set standards, regulate practices and facilitate human interactions (as in contract law). We find many of these functions performed in medical law.

Branches of law

Medical law has grown from lots of other branches of law to become an area of law in its own right. If one thinks of law as a large tree, there are numerous branches, some entwining with one another, others growing away from the other branches, creating distinct areas of law. One basic distinction is between public law, which concerns my relationship with the state (as in criminal law), and private law, which concerns my relationship with other individuals (as in contract law). A more helpful distinction is between civil law and criminal law, although even this distinction can be hard to draw . . .

Civil law (and tort law)

Basically, civil law differs from criminal law because it usually involves compensation rather than punishment by the state. The most important area of civil law for doctors is **tort law**, which encompasses a variety of legal wrongs or 'torts'. Tort law is notoriously difficult to define, but one can think of it as concerned with the protection of interests. Thus, tort law includes defamation (my interest in my good character), trespass to land (my interest in my property) and, particularly important in healthcare, trespass to the person (my interest in my bodily integrity) and negligence (my interest in being treated carefully or reasonably).

Civil law has its own procedures, outcomes and terminology. Some key words and concepts are: The **claimant** (once known as 'the plaintiff'), usually the patient in healthcare cases . . . **sues** (or 'brings an action against') . . . the **defendant**, who is alleged to have committed a **civil wrong**, like a tort (this is usually a health professional or their employer). If the claimant wins her case, the defendant is found . . . **liable**. In a **tort action**, this means that the claimant is awarded . . . **damages**, a financial sum, which the defendant must pay (or, more often, which the defendant's employer or insurer must pay). As civil law is concerned with compensation, the sum is intended to put the claimant in the position they would have been but for the wrongful actions of the defendant. Many of these terms are specific to civil law; criminal law has its own words and traditions and lawyers must learn to keep the two separate. (For example, signs declaring that 'Trespassers will be prosecuted' are inaccurate because trespassing land is a civil matter, whereas prosecution is a criminal matter!)

Criminal law

Criminal law, unlike civil law, is primarily a matter for the state and differs because the guilty defendant will be punished. Some key words and concepts are: The **victim** of a crime has his case investigated by the police, who pass the case onto . . . the **prosecutor**, who is usually someone working for the **Crown Prosecution Service**. She prosecutes . . . the **defendant**, the person accused of committing the crime. If the prosecution 'fails', the defendant is **acquitted** (found innocent). However, if the prosecution 'succeeds', the defendant is found **guilty**, which results in . . . a **conviction**, which results in . . . **punishment**, which can take various forms, such as a **fine**, a **probation order** (involving, eg, counselling or treatment) or, at worst, **imprisonment**.

It is important to recognise that it is never obvious whether something is, or should be, a crime. We might all think that actions such as murder or theft should be punishable but it remains up to the particular state to declare that this will be the case. So it is not the nature of the action (or failure to act) that makes something a crime – rather, it is the legal consequences that can flow from it. For example, if I touched a patient without his consent, I might have committed the crimes of assault or battery and may, in the worst case, be imprisoned. However, that same non-consensual touching is also a civil wrong: the tort of trespass to the person, which means that I could also be sued and might have to pay out in compensation. Note that this is an additional legal wrong, so a particular action can in theory lead to my coming before two different courts.

Sources of law

We are discussing here the English legal system, which is shorthand for the law governing England and Wales (although Wales has also gained some local law-making powers in recent years). Scotland and Northern Ireland have their own legal systems, as will other states (or 'jurisdictions'), and if you are practising in another jurisdiction it will be worth familiarising yourself with the basic principles of law relevant to your practice. Focusing on England and Wales, however, there are four important sources of law.

Common law

Common law is otherwise known as **case law**, which is the law developed by the judges in their judgments (or rulings) on particular cases. The judges are guided by the theory and **rules of precedent**, which means they are bound by previous rulings that set 'precedents'. This essentially means that they must take into account similar cases decided in the past, particularly those decided in the highest courts (such as the House of Lords).

This area of judge-made law is important because there will be situations where Parliament has not enacted a law and it falls to the judges to plug the gap. Equally, judges must sometimes interpret laws that Parliament has passed. One such example involved the Abortion Act 1967. A secretary declined to type a referral letter for a termination, claiming that the right to conscientiously object to participation in an abortion protected her refusal. The judges looked at the word 'participation' and decided that the secretary was not covered, as she was not sufficiently involved in the procedure.

Judges will always be needed to plug the gaps and interpret the law because, as you may already be aware, the law is not complete and is not always clear. But this is not to say that there are not areas where the law is certain, as we shall see when we turn to some of the key principles of healthcare law.

Statute law

A statute is an **Act of Parliament** (or just an 'Act'), which is a document written and passed by Parliament designed to tackle a particular problem or area of practice. An Act is known as a, Bill, before it is passed, by which we mean accepted by the legislature, ie the House of Commons and the House of Lords. Once it has been passed, an Act can be referred to as **primary legislation**.

Many Acts are relevant to healthcare, such as the Abortion Act 1967, the Human Tissue Act 2004 and the Human Fertilisation and Embryology Act 1990. The title usually conveys the area(s) covered by the Act and the year is the year in which the Act was passed. Sometimes there is a delay between the Act being passed and its coming into force, ie its application in practice. This makes sense because some Acts, particularly in healthcare, require people to be trained in the new law and regulatory bodies to be created. The Human Tissue Act 2004 is one such example, as it will come into force in 2006, by which time a new Human Tissue Authority will have been created. Acts are divided into numbered sections (denoted by 's.') and subsections (denoted by 'ss.'), and sometimes contain 'Schedules' at the end, which can be helpful in understanding the words used in the rest of the Act.

Some Acts are rather like parents, since they spawn, children, in the form of **secondary legislation**. Such secondary legislation may be known as **regulations** or 'statutory instruments'. For example, in s. 45 and Schedule 2 of the Human Fertilisation and Embryology Act 1990, the Secretary of State was empowered to issue new regulations. Hence, the Human Fertilisation and Embryology (Research Purposes) Regulations 2001 were passed, which amended the parent Act so as to allow the cloning of human embryos (under 14 days' gestation) for research purposes. Sometimes these regulations can be more important in practice than the parent Act. For example, a regulation issued in 1991 under the Abortion Act is useful to medical professionals since it sets out the pro forma for declaring that an abortion is lawful.

European Convention of Human Rights Law

The European Convention on Human Rights and Fundamental Freedoms is a convention to which individual European states may commit themselves. The UK has done so and this means that any citizen who feels that the State has violated their rights may take a claim before the European Court of Human Rights (ECHR) in Strasbourg.

This used to mean that the individual had to go through all the English courts first (using English law principles) before bringing a human rights claim. The situation changed in 2000, when the Human Rights Act 1998 came into force. This Act essentially brings the ECHR rights directly into English law. The individual can still go to Strasbourg, but they can also now rely on human rights arguments in this jurisdiction (as the Government stated at the time, the Act 'brings rights back home'). Nowadays, UK Acts and rulings must be compatible with these rights. An individual can therefore now use human rights arguments in English courts, in addition to any arguments based on pre-existing English law. The Act still only applies at the state level: it says that 'public authorities' must respect human rights. This actually means that all doctors must respect human rights, because they will be working in the NHS (a state body) and/or will be registered with the GMC (which is empowered by the state to regulate doctors).

European Union law

European Union (EU), or European Community, law differs from the law of the ECHR. It is most concerned with trade between member states of the EU. It has its own legal processes and court system, with the European Court of Justice sitting in Luxembourg.

Although it may not appear as directly relevant to healthcare practice as the ECHR, there are areas in which the influence of the EU is significant: the Data Protection Act 1998, for example, resulted from EU law, as did changes to the way in which research ethics committees are regulated. Furthermore, its influence can be seen in the laws relating to developments in biotechnology, the regulation of pharmaceutical products and even the free movement of individuals between European states to receive healthcare.

Professional obligations: General Medical Council

In your day-to-day practice it will rarely be necessary for you to consult directly the laws coming from the courts, Parliament and Europe. Rather, it will usually suffice for you to look at the guidance and codes of practice issued by the GMC, the British Medical Association (BMA), your insurer, the Royal Colleges and the Department of Health. What roles do such bodies play and what is the status of their guidance?

If we focus on the GMC, it regulates the medical profession in the UK, maintains the medical registers of doctors seeking to practise medicine in the UK and provides guidance and standards for practice (eg *Duties of a Doctor* and *Good Medical Practice*) and education (eg *Tomorrow's Doctors*). It has the power to discipline doctors if necessary, and to suspend or even remove them from the register (which we call 'being struck off').

Historically, the British Courts have given substantial power to the GMC in allowing doctors to make decisions about the consequences of poor practice. This is partly because the courts accept that most judges are not medically experienced. It is for the same reason that in a negligence case, a medical expert or experts will be called on to advise the court on events that are in dispute.

Although the GMC is given considerable autonomy in dealing with doctors, in some cases doctors may find themselves coming before both the GMC and the British legal system. Doctors who are brought before the GMC are investigated by Fitness to Practise committees. The role of Fitness to Practise committees has been formalised and is becoming more structured as a result of Dame Janet Smith's recommendations in the fifth Shipman Inquiry Report.

Turning to the guidance and codes issued by the GMC, these can be seen as a type of 'quasi-law'. Some of the GMC guidance may indeed take the form of rules, which it would be foolhardy to ignore, given the GMC's role as your professional regulator. Moreover, the guidance sometimes plugs gaps in the law that the courts have not yet had the opportunity to address, and it is also the case that, on occasion, the courts will openly endorse the GMC's position. For example, this has occurred in the context of maintaining confidentiality. Such guidance can therefore influence the law and will itself have been drafted in the light of any law that already exists.

British judicial system

There are many different courts in the UK, hearing various types of case. Courts of first instance, where cases are first heard, include the Crown Court (for serious criminal matters), the County Court and the Magistrates' courts. However, many cases in medical law begin in the High Court, specifically in that branch of the High Court known as the 'Family Division'. Here, it is usual for there to be one judge, such as Mr Justice Johnson (Johnson J). The head of the Family Division of the High Court is called the President (eg Dame Elizabeth Butler-Sloss P).

If either party is dissatisfied with the initial ruling, it has the opportunity to appeal to a higher court. In medical law, the Court of Appeal is often the next in the chain and it comprises three judges, eg Lord Justice Ward (Ward LJ). The head of the Court of Appeal is called the Master of the Rolls (eg Donaldson MR). A system of majority rule operates, such that if there is a split opinion, the majority's decision sets the precedent. (However, law is not static and future judges might come to prefer the opinion of the minority as better representing the law.)

From the Court of Appeal there can be an appeal to the House of Lords, if the case is on a matter of particular legal importance. Here there are five judges, such as Lord Goff (Goff L). The head of the House of Lords is the Lord Chancellor (eg Irvine LC). Note that when we refer to the House of Lords here we mean it in its judicial role (ie composed only of judges hearing a case), as opposed to its separate role as a House of Parliament.

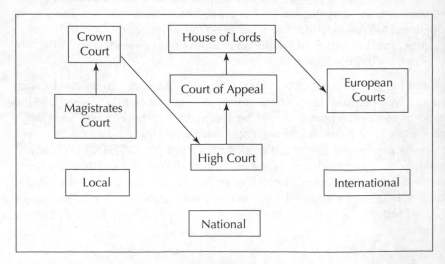

As already mentioned, there are also the European courts, and these can be the courts of last resort in cases that involve points of European law. The figure shows the organisation of the court system in England and Wales as a general guide to the different levels of the judicial process. This will vary in each jurisdiction and we will not attempt to provide a comprehensive overview here.

Some key legal concepts

Competence/capacity

Broadly speaking, a patient who is competent (has capacity) is entitled to make their own decision about treatment or non-treatment. If the patient is 16 or over, you are to presume that they are competent. If you have doubts, however, you may test a patient's competence by asking:

- Can she comprehend and retain the information?
- Does she believe it?
- Has she weighed it in the balance to arrive at a choice?

Note that this assessment is a matter for the doctor responsible for the patient's care; psychiatrists and the like are not needed, but can be called on to help make the assessment. If the patient is competent, you may accept her consent; furthermore, if she is 18 or over and she competently refuses treatment, you must honour that refusal.

The situation is a little different for under-16s. The main question to ask is, 'Is the minor of sufficient understanding and intelligence to comprehend what is proposed, any risks/benefits or alternatives etc?' If you feel that he or she is, and the patient consents, you may proceed with treatment and you do not need to ask someone else (such as a parent) to consent. However, even the competent minor (someone under 18) does not have the right to 'veto' treatment. In other words, if a patient under 16 refuses to consent, you may still obtain consent or authorisation for the treatment from someone such as a parent or a court.

Consent to and refusal of treatment

A legally valid consent requires:

- a competent patient
- a voluntary decision – free from coercion, force or fraud
- sufficient information – you must have informed the patient in 'broad terms' of the nature of the procedure and must go some way to ensuring that the consent is appropriately informed. English law does not (yet) require fully 'informed consent', but you must answer questions truthfully and disclose information about material (significant) risks.

You should also ensure that you observe any legal boundaries to the consent. For example, a patient may be competent, informed and deciding voluntarily that they want assistance in suicide but as this is currently unlawful, and you are not entitled to act on their request. There may also be additional requirements attached to some procedures, such as the need for the consent to be in writing if the patient is seeking assisted reproduction.

Best interests

If the patient is not competent to consent to treatment, it may still be given, provided that you act in the patient's 'best interests'. This calculation must take account of both medical matters and wider issues, such as any relevant familial, spiritual or cultural interests that the patient may have. With children, parents (or, strictly speaking, those with 'parental responsibility') can help you make this assessment; adults cannot yet appoint proxy decision-makers, although the situation looks likely to change under the proposed Mental Capacity Bill.

Confidentiality

Maintaining patient confidentiality is important, not only ethically but also legally, as an aggrieved patient can bring an action for breach of confidence. Sometimes disclosure may be justified, such as in the 'public interest', to protect others from the risk of serious harm (such as child abuse). You must make sure, however, that you only disclose the information to people who genuinely need to know (eg the police or your colleagues). If the disclosure was unlawful, the patient may be awarded damages or be granted an injunction (which stops 'publication'); moreover, your employer and the GMC are unlikely to look kindly on serious breaches of confidentiality.

Clinical negligence

Clinical negligence is, as we have seen, a tort. In order to succeed, the claimant (usually the patient) must prove that they:

- were owed a duty of care . . .
- which was breached, ie the care was not of a sufficient standard. This is often governed by the **Bolam standard** (from the case *Bolam v Friern Hospital Management Committee* [1957] 1 WLR 582), which holds that a doctor is not negligent if he or she has acted in accordance with responsible medical practice. The body of thought (or practice) must still have a logical basis, however, and it remains for the court to say whether a particular practice is sufficiently careful . . .
- which caused the patient harm.

If the patient succeeds, they may be awarded damages.

Legal research and writing

Although you will not normally be expected to know how to research and write on matters of law, there may be occasions when you will have to do so, such as when working on an SSM or studying for a BSc or postgraduate qualification in healthcare law. The following sections offer you a few pointers to help you get started.

Inside the law library

Many universities in the UK offer degrees in law and most of these will have a library devoted to legal materials. However, once you are inside, the material can be difficult to locate and comprehend. We very much recommend speaking with the law librarians, who should be able to point you to such useful resources as:

- A **law dictionary** – Although there has been a move away from the use of Latin and other specialist terminology in recent times, there will still be legal terms and concepts that are unfamiliar or have a meaning rather different from the one familiar to non-lawyers. A legal dictionary can help clarify points of confusion.
- A **legal citator** – A text which helps explain some of the acronyms and abbreviations used (for example in case law reports).
- **Case law reports** – There are various series of reports, which contain the full text of judgments delivered in the courts (particularly the higher courts). Each report opens with a brief summary of the main points of the ruling (this part is known as the 'headnote' and can help guide your reading of the full ruling).
- **Statute books** – These contain the full text of Acts of Parliament and, where relevant, should also point you to any subsequent amendments to the Act, so that you have the most up-to-date account of the law. There are also textbooks published periodically which collect together all the Acts relevant to a particular legal topic, eg criminal law.
- **Legal journals** – These are usually specific to an area of law (eg medical law, as in the *Medical Law Review*) and will contain academic articles on particular topics in addition to what are known as 'case notes' or 'case commentaries'. The latter can be very useful, as they summarise recent rulings, place them in the context of the law to date, and offer assessments of the rights and wrongs of the judge's opinion. These can be helpful in preparing for assignments in law (see below).
- **Legal textbooks** – These are usually the best place to start. There are plenty of textbooks devoted to medical law and healthcare law and

they will usually be titled accordingly. Be careful, though, to use the most recent editions of the textbooks, as the law is constantly evolving.

■ **Internet** – In addition to the above resources, you will also find a wealth of legal material on the Internet. Caution is always advisable when using this as a research tool, but there are some very good search engines available, such as Westlaw, which tracks developments in cases and features those academic publications that offer case commentaries.

Types of question

Whether working in examination conditions or on a piece of assessed coursework, law students tend to be asked to tackle two types of question:

An essay question

Either a direct question is posed ('Should physician-assisted suicide be legalised?') or the student is invited to analyse a proposition ('Legalising physician-assisted suicide would be dangerous. Discuss.'). The question will usually focus on one or two areas of the law and the best answers will introduce the position taken by the student, offer arguments and deal with counter-arguments, and then conclude with a summary of the arguments and the position taken. A logical structure is recommended but, apart from these tips, there is rarely a 'right' answer – there are only well-argued and less well-argued approaches to the issues.

A problem question

This type of question will be more familiar to you from your medical studies, as it presents a relatively detailed account of a situation on which the student is asked to advise (often as if he or she were a lawyer in the case). Virtually every part of the question will have been included for a reason, so there will be something worthy of comment in every paragraph. Here, the better answers will again proceed logically and will not only offer a positive case for or against something (eg 'Dr Smith is liable in negligence because . . .') but will also acknowledge those aspects that are legally uncertain or even inconsistent. Inconsistency arises from time to time, not only because judges hear lots of cases, but also because law is all about interpretation of 'similar' cases and principles; a smart barrister may therefore be able to convince the court that his client's case differs from an established precedent.

Whichever type of question you encounter, the best advice is the most obvious: read the question and answer it! Law teachers still encounter students who re-interpret the question to ask what they would prefer to write about, rather than what the question is asking them to write about. There is also an important health warning associated with assessments in law (and, indeed, the law more generally): there is not always a clear answer. Again, this is due to the need for interpretation and can also be attributed to the fact that English law proceeds on an adversarial basis, ie there are two parties 'battling' to prove that their view of the facts and the law is the right one. If you treat such assignments as an exercise in persuasion, you are on the right lines and it can be very rewarding to persuade your tutor of the legal force of your arguments, provided of course that you argue within the parameters of the law as it stands.

Referencing legal materials

In referring to legal material, there are some conventions to observe, particularly when writing about Acts of Parliament and the common law.

Acts of Parliament

Acts of Parliament may be stated in the main text or in a note (footnote or endnote). For example:

The welfare principle is contained in s. 1(3) of the Children Act 1989, which states that . . .

Rulings/precedents

Rulings are a little trickier. You may put the citation in the main text or in a note. For example:

In *Smith v Jones* [2005] 1 QB 305, McDonald J held that a patient . . .

or

In *Smith v Jones*[5], McDonald J held that a patient . . .

With the latter approach, footnote (or endnote) number 5 will then contain the citation, ie [2005] 1 QB 305.

In both examples, you read the citation as follows:

'Smith *and* Jones, reported in 2005, in the first volume of the Queen's Bench Law Reports at page 305'. The page number is the page on which the text of the ruling starts; if you are making explicit reference to a particular page, this may be done as follows:

[2005] 1 QB 305, 311 (or 'at 311') . . .

Whichever method you prefer, you need not provide the full reference more than once. As long as it is clear which case you are referring to, you may abbreviate. For example:

Smith v Jones [2005] 1 QB 305 (hereafter *Smith*) . . .

You may then refer to *Smith* for the remainder of the assignment.

The case above was a hypothetical example, based on a real series of law reports. There are lots of these and you are advised to seek advice if you need to find one. Some examples of actual case reports include:

Re A (Children)(Conjoined Twins: Surgical Separation) [2000] 4 All ER 961: reported in 2000, in the fourth volume of the All England Law Reports at page 961. This was the conjoined twins ruling mentioned earlier in the chapter, where the children are referred to as 'A', in order to preserve anonymity (note also that 'Jodie' and 'Mary' were not their real names).

Re B (Adult: Refusal of Medical Treatment) [2002] 2 All ER 449: reported in 2002, in the second volume of the All England Law Reports at page 449. This was the case of 'Ms B', the paralysed woman who did not want to receive artificial ventilation.

Bolam v Friern Hospital Management Committee [1957] 1 WLR 582: reported in 1957, in the first volume of the Weekly Law Reports at page 582. This was the case of Mr Bolam, which set the precedent governing the standard of care in clinical negligence cases.

Chapter Five
THE CASES

HOW TO USE THIS CHAPTER

This chapter contains a variety of cases that draw their inspiration from actual events. You may like to discuss how you would approach these situations and why, either individually or in small groups. Medical teachers may wish to use the cases to stimulate discussion of generic ethical or medico-legal issues.

We do not necessarily give all the solutions to these cases, but that is because sometimes there *are* no right answers – or none that are more right than your own. What this chapter *will* do is give you some key information that you need to know, in terms of laws and important ethical theories. This will help you to be able to reach decisions, both within the context of the following cases and in your own practice. More importantly, it will allow you to justify and explain your position with reference to well-reasoned principles.

Each case is followed by a summary at the end. In addition a reading list which can be referenced for more information, or greater detail on existing information. Within the cases, points for discussion and revision have been marked with the following symbols:

✿ **Discussion point** and ✸ **Revision point**

Most of the cases deal with a range of different issues. If you want to revise particular themes, refer to the overleaf list, which shows which cases cover which aspects. This list of themes was drawn up by the Consensus Group of Teachers of Medical Ethics and Law, as a core curriculum in medical ethics and law for medical schools in the UK (Consensus Group of Teachers of Medical Ethics and Law in UK Medical Schools. Teaching medical ethics and law within medical education: a model for the UK core curriculum. *Journal of Medical Ethics* 1998; 24: 188–92).

Core content

- Informed consent and refusal of treatment
  Cases: 2–5, 8, 13, 19, 23

- The clinical relationship: truthfulness, trust, and good communication
  Cases: 1–25

- Confidentiality
  Cases: 1, 2, 4, 7, 10, 12–15, 22

- Medical research
  Cases: 8, 9, 16, 21–23

- Human reproduction and the new genetics
  Cases: 14, 16

- Children
  Cases: 4, 5, 8, 11, 14–16

- Mental disorders and disabilities
  Cases: 3, 4, 12, 13, 17

- Life, death, dying and killing
  Cases: 2, 3, 5, 8, 9, 13, 14, 16, 17, 24

- Vulnerabilities created by the duties of doctors and medical students
  Cases: 1, 3, 5, 6–11, 13–24

- Resource allocation
  Cases: 2, 8, 9, 11, 16, 17, 21, 23

- Rights including the Human Rights Act 1998
  Cases: 2–5, 7–9, 11–14, 16, 17, 19, 22, 23, 25

Issues raised in each case

Case 1: The DVLA and the epileptic patient
- Driver and Vehicle Licensing Authority (DVLA)
- Patient's versus society's interests
- Breaching confidentiality

Case 2: Withdrawal of ventilation
- Advance directives/statements (also known as 'living wills')
- Consent
- 'Do not attempt resuscitation' (DNAR) orders
- Quality-of-life issues

- Acts and omissions and the doctrine of 'double effect'
- The cases of Diane Pretty and Leslie Burke
- Communication issues within the healthcare team
- Allocation of resources

Case 3: The incompetent adult and advance directives
- Advance directives
- Relatives
- Proxy consent and the Mental Capacity Act 2005
- Adults with Incapacity Act (Scotland) 2000
- The law on euthanasia in the Netherlands – recent developments

Case 4: The 15-year-old with diabetes
- Duty of care
- Competence and age of medical consent

Case 5: The 15-year-old Jehovah's Witness
- Refusing treatment – competent minors
- Considering 'best interests'

Case 6: The negligent surgeon
- Negligence
- Reporting poor clinical practice
- Doctors and their families requiring medical treatment

Case 7: The sick colleague
- Looking after each other – ethics of working in a team
- Risks to patients
- Stealing from the hospital
- Breaking the law

Case 8: Death of a child
- Death certificates
- Cremation forms
- Notifying the coroner
- Post-mortem examinations
- Holding an inquest

Case 9: Organ donation
- Organ donation and transplantation
- Respecting cultural and religious beliefs
- Reform of the law relating to organ donation

Case 10: Confidentiality and duty of care
- Consent to investigations
- Duty of care
- Breaching confidentiality

Case 11: The young mother
- Controversial treatments
- Prevention versus treatment
- Refusing consent for minors
- Relationship of trust

Case 12: The anorexic patient
- Confidentiality
- Eating disorders and the Mental Health Act
- Assessment and the Mental Health Act
- Compulsory treatment and the Mental Health Act
- Autonomy and paternalism
- Mental Health Act reform

Case 13: The suicidal patient
- Suicide
- Treatment restrictions under the Mental Health Act
- Doctors with mental disorders

Case 14: Abortion
- Truth-telling and confidentiality
- Conflicting rights
- Abortion Act 1967
- When does life begin?

Case 15: Sexual abuse of minors
- Investigation of allegations
- Confidentiality and privacy
- Consent from minors
- Children Act 1989

Case 16: Bone marrow transplant and fertility treatment
- Fertility treatment
- 'Motives' for childbearing
- Human Fertilisation and Embryology Act 1990
- Embryo selection ('designer babies')
- Apocalypse now?
- Therapeutic cloning
- Resource allocation and rationing

Case 17: Scarce resources
- Rationing
- Allocation of resources
- Quality-Adjusted Life-Years (QALYs)

Case 18: Relationships with patients
- Personal relationships with patients
- Professional responsibilities of medical students

Case 19: Performing intimate examinations
- Changing patient attitudes
- Investigation of allegations and rumours
- Bullying and harassment
- Obtaining consent for examinations
- Students in operating theatres as assistants
- Patients who lack competence
- Liability when no consent is obtained
- Admission of errors to patients and apologies

Case 20: Professional courtesy and foul play
- Cheating and plagiarism
- Reporting concerns about colleagues
- Queue jumping

Case 21: Is there such a thing as a free lunch?
- Professional obligations
- Autonomous decisions – the choice of individuals

Case 22: Publication ethics, data protection and freedom of information
- Publication ethics

Case 23: Medicine in the developing world – elective ethics?
- Professional obligations for medical students
- Universality of ethical principles – global research, global ethics
- Doctors and torture
- Consequentialism versus deontology

Case 24: Medical practice in the post-Shipman era
- Keeping tabs? (Professional regulation)
- Gifts from patients

Case 25: Medicine in the age of the Human Rights Act
- Human Rights Act 1998

CASE 1: THE DVLA AND THE EPILEPTIC PATIENT

Issues

Driver and Vehicle Licensing Authority
Patient's versus society's interests
Breaching confidentiality

You are a recently appointed specialist registrar (SpR) in neurology. Following investigations during a recent hospital stay, one of your patients, Mr Evans, a middle-aged taxi driver, was diagnosed as having epilepsy. Before he left the hospital you advised him to stop driving, and that he should contact the DVLA to make them aware of his epilepsy. Although this meant the end of his livelihood, he undertook to do so.

One month later he is due to attend an out-patient appointment at your clinic. On the morning of the clinic, one of the specialist nurses (a neighbour of the patient) tells you that he has continued to drive. Furthermore, she believes that he has not yet told his wife and family of the diagnosis – let alone his employer or the DVLA.

- **What are your responsibilities in this case?**
- **Would you tell:**
  - **the DVLA?**
  - **the family?**
  - **the police?**
  - **the employer?**
- **Should you take any action?**

Use this page to write down your own ideas

Driver and Vehicle Licensing Authority

It is the patient's responsibility to inform the DVLA of health conditions that might cause them to pose a risk to themselves or other road users by driving. These conditions include:

- psychiatric disorders, eg chronic schizophrenia
- neurological disorders, eg epilepsy
- diabetes mellitus
- visual problems, eg monocular vision, diplopia.

Informing the DVLA does not necessarily lead to automatic suspension. The DVLA will assess whether the condition is severe enough to warrant a driving ban, either indefinitely or for a limited period. Certain other medical conditions, such as cardiovascular disorders and procedures (eg myocardial infarction or angioplasty) require driving restrictions, although the DVLA need not be notified. Doctors should inform their patients if they will need to abstain from driving for a period of time for medical reasons.

If a patient neglects their responsibility and continues to drive then the doctor is morally and professionally obliged to take action (see GMC guidance[1] on confidentiality for specific advice relating to this situation). In the first instance you should try to persuade patients to tell the DVLA themselves. In this case, the patient should be persuaded to tell his family the diagnosis too, as this is in his best interests, eg they could be educated to provide appropriate care should he have a seizure at home. However, if the patient still refuses what can you do?

✿ Doctors are bound by a duty of confidentiality that covers any information they acquire in their professional capacity. However, this is not an unqualified or absolute duty.

✿ What is confidentiality? What does it mean to the patient and has it been explained to them? What does it mean to you as a doctor?

✿ Telling the DVLA constitutes a breach of the patient's confidentiality. On what ethical grounds could you justify such action?

Patient's versus society's interests

To justify *legally* breaching confidentiality, reference is made to the interpretation of a case (*W v Egdell* [1989] 1 All ER 1089) in which the court held that where there is a serious risk of physical harm to an identifiable individual or individuals, a doctor can (but not necessarily must) breach confidentiality. In order to breach confidentiality, not doing so would have to pose a risk to the patient or to others. In the circumstances of this case the doctor can probably be satisfied that this is the case and is justified in breaching confidentiality. However, breaches of confidentiality should be on a 'need to know' basis only, with need being defined as the minimum necessary to protect the safety of others. Therefore telling the DVLA would therefore be justifiable, but telling the local population, on the basis that they might get into the patient's taxi, would not be.

✿ If this is so, why not just go ahead and tell the DVLA yourself in the first place, instead of depending on a perhaps unreliable patient to do so? What effect would this have on patient care?

✿ If doctors had no code of confidentiality and patients knew that bodies such as the DVLA, insurance companies, the police and the government could have unlimited access to their health information, how would this change medical practice?

✿ What is the point of having a requirement to maintain patient confidentiality?

✿ In this case, you are told by a third party that the patient is continuing to drive. What happens in situations where you do not have access to such information? How can you be sure that the patient will stop driving? How far can/should you go in trying to find out whether they have stopped driving?

Writing to the GP, explaining that you have discussed with the patient the need to inform the DVLA, is an obvious first line. Doctors are justified in sharing medical information with other healthcare professionals involved in providing care for their patient, thus ensuring optimal continuity of care for the patient. It is good practice always to tell the patient that you will write a letter to their GP with a summary of your meeting and the results of any investigations done so that you keep them informed. Better still, many hospital doctors these days write a letter to the patient, copied to the GP. However, patients do have the right to ask that even medical personnel are not told certain information.

The guidelines for medical students are slightly different. As a medical student you may well receive information that is pertinent to a patient's care but which the patient asks you to keep from the rest of the team, eg non-compliance with treatment. As a student you cannot offer complete confidentiality, particularly where to do so would be to compromise the patient's care. You must explain that confidentiality is within the healthcare team and as a student, you would like them to discuss what they have told you with someone more senior. If the patient refuses, you should explain that you will have to discuss it with your seniors and why this is the case.

✿ Would you be happy to pass the buck to the GP, ie assume that the GP will make sure the patient tells the DVLA or, if necessary, tell the DVLA themselves? Do you feel that both you and the GP share this responsibility? Would you feel responsible if the patient caused an accident because he had an epileptic fit while driving?

Breaching confidentiality

If a patient feels that a breach of confidence was not justified they can make a complaint. Although the patient also has the right to take legal action, this can be costly and may not result in the award of any monetary compensation even if the court finds in favour of the claimant. If the GMC determines that the doctor was not justified in breaching patient confidentiality, then the doctor could be liable for professional misconduct in the most serious cases and could be struck off the medical register.

The GMC gives details of several possible situations which would allow a doctor to disclose patient information.[1] The areas are summarised below:

- If the patient gives written consent, eg for research.
- If disclosure would be in the patient's best interests but it is impracticable to obtain consent, eg sharing information with others providing care to an incapacitous patient. This includes other healthcare professionals but may, exceptionally, also include a close relative, eg in cases of dementia.
- If disclosure would be in the public interest:
  - if required to do so by a court order or Act of Parliament, eg notifiable diseases, Prevention of Terrorism legislation
  - if failure to breach poses a risk of death or serious harm to the patient or others, eg child abuse, rape, serious violence.

Although the law is broadly in agreement with GMC guidance, the legal standpoint is less clearly defined. Legally, doctors are justified in breaching confidentiality *without* the patient's consent in the following circumstances:

- When ordered to do so by law:
  - by a court order
  - under Acts of Parliament, eg in the case of notifiable diseases.
- When it is in the public interest.

✿ What is the difference between a *duty* to breach confidentiality and an *entitlement* to do so?

Breaching confidentiality 'in the public interest' is a very difficult decision to make and may ultimately be down to the courts to determine. In an English case (*Hill v Chief Constable for West Yorkshire* [1987] 2 WLR 1126) it was decided that there was no **duty** to inform in the public interest.

However, a different view was taken in a famous American case (*Tarasoff v Regents of the University of California,* 131, Cal Rptr 14 Cal S Ct of CA (1976)). Mr Poddar, a male college student, told a university psychiatrist during a therapy session that he wanted to kill a fellow student (Tatiana Tarasoff) who had been refusing his advances. The doctor informed the campus police, who then assessed the man but released him when he appeared rational and promised to stay away from Ms Tarasoff. Poddar then went ahead and murdered Tarasoff on her return to campus from holiday. The parents sued the university for failure to inform their daughter of the risk. The US court found the doctor liable for negligence because he had not warned Tatiana of the potential risk to her life. The judge stated 'the protective privilege ends where the public peril begins'.

In the UK it is unlikely that a similar decision would have been reached since courts in the UK are reluctant to make one person liable for the crime committed by another (this was confirmed in the cases of *Clunis v Camden and Islington Health Authority* [1998] QB 978 and *Palmer v Tees HA* [2000] PIQR 1).

The GMC requires that confidentiality should be maintained even after the patient's death (see Section 5 of *Confidentiality: Protecting and Providing Information*[1]; the law, on the other hand, may not require this. Note that solicitors and police officers have no special right to confidential information. Disclose information only if you decide that it is justified under one of the above conditions.

Breaching confidentiality to relatives

Disclosing information to relatives is sometimes difficult to judge. If it can be assumed that the patient would give consent for information to be disclosed to their family, the doctor can probably go ahead and impart information to the relatives without consulting the patient, who may be either too sick or unable to communicate. This should be done tactfully however, and confidential information should never be given over the phone. However, if the patient has expressly forbidden such communication, this wish should be respected. The patient has a right to maintain confidentiality even when the doctor considers it not to be in the patient's best interests. Therefore, in the case of the epileptic driver, it may well be in his best interests for his family to know his diagnosis, but if he states that he does not want them to know, you cannot tell them.

Conditions when doctors are <u>legally required</u> to breach confidentiality

- If required to do so by a court of law. Judges will do their best to ensure that any breaches of confidentiality are kept to those relevant to the trial:
    - doctors can be subpoenaed (ordered) to give evidence in court
    - doctors (unlike lawyers) may not refuse to answer questions or withhold evidence.
- Prevention of Terrorism Act 1989:
    - doctors (like any member of the public) must take the initiative to inform the police of any information regarding terrorist activities.
- Police and Criminal Evidence Act 1984:
    - doctors must answer police questions or provide any evidence requested by them
    - police can have access to medical records but must abide by certain conditions.
- The Public Health (Control of Disease) Act 1984.
    - notifiable diseases include cholera, plague, smallpox, relapsing fever and typhus (note that HIV/AIDS is not a notifiable disease)
    - other diseases can fall under this Act should an epidemic occur.
- Accidents at work.
- Incidents of food poisoning.
- Life events:
    - doctors must report births, deaths and abortions.
- Misuse of Drugs Act:
    - doctors must report details of known drug addicts.
- Health administration:
    - doctors must provide information on request to the Department of Health, regional and district health authorities among others.

✩ Can you see any discrepancies in these conditions? It has been argued that people with HIV will be deterred from seeking medical treatment if it is a notifiable disease and that it is therefore not in the public interest to make it notifiable. However, details of drug users must be reported.

Under the Police and Criminal Evidence Act 1984, if the police contact the doctor, the doctor must answer their questions and provide evidence if necessary. However, if the doctor knows that a patient has, or is about to, commit a criminal offence, they are under no legal obligation to take the initiative to contact the police.

It could be argued that all citizens have a moral duty to society to prevent and report any crime. The law is excusing doctors from this duty because it believes that there may be situations when it can be in the public interest for doctors to maintain patient confidentiality rather than for certain criminals to be convicted. Moreover, a lot of the information doctors may receive is in the context of their therapeutic relationship rather than as 'citizens'.

The exception to this rule is if the information pertains to terrorist activities. Section 18 of the Prevention of Terrorism Act 1989 states anyone (including doctors) in possession of such information must *take the initiative* to disclose it to the police.

If in doubt, seek legal advice from your defence organisation!

Summary

- Doctors are bound by a duty of confidentiality to their patients.
- Deciding whether to breach confidentiality requires a careful balance of risk of harm to the patient versus risk of physical harm to others.
- The law requires doctors to breach confidentiality in certain situations.
- It is the patient's responsibility to inform bodies such as the DVLA or their employer but, if the patient refuses, the doctor must take action.

Reading

- DVLA. www.dvla.gov.uk – go to driver's information, and medical rules.
- Epilepsy Action. www.epilepsy.org.uk – go to information, then driving.
- General Medical Council. *Confidentiality: Protecting and Providing Information.* London: GMC, 2000: section 5 and appendix 2.
- Montauk L, Morrison V. Crime, confidentiality, and clinical judgment. *Lancet* 364 (Suppl 1).
- Shorvon S. Epilepsy and driving. *BMJ* 1995; 310: 885–6.

Reference

1. General Medical Council. *Confidentiality: Protecting and Providing Information.* London: GMC, 2000.

CASE 2: WITHDRAWAL OF VENTILATION

Issues

Advance directives/statements ('living wills')
Consent
'Do not attempt resuscitation' (DNAR) orders
Quality-of-life issues
Acts and omissions and the doctrine of 'double effect'
The cases of Diane Pretty and Leslie Burke
Communication issues within the healthcare team
Allocation of resources

You are a senior house officer (SHO) working in general medicine. A 19-year-old man was diagnosed with motor neurone disease when he was 17. The disease was very aggressive and rapidly progressive.

At a time when his communication was already limited he made it known that he wished to state in an advance directive that should he suffer a cardiopulmonary arrest he would not want to be resuscitated.

He did suffer a respiratory arrest and was ventilated. You were part of the crash team that attended him. The nurses on the ward did inform the team leader of the advance directive but were told not to interfere.

- **Would you have resuscitated and ventilated this man?**
- **What should be done now that he is on a ventilator?**

Use this page to write down your own ideas

Advance directives/statements (living wills)

An advance directive (or living will) is a statement (usually a written document) in which a person stipulates the circumstances under which they would or would not wish to receive medical treatment (or to what extent they would want to receive active treatment). It is intended to provide directions if and when a situation arises when they are not competent to make their own decisions. In discussing this case, one would probably look at the situation that the patient was in when the advance directive was made, and consider the validity of that directive.

✿ How do *you* feel about advance directives? What are their pros and cons? Should they be legally binding?

✿ Would you be happy to act according to an advance directive if an unconscious patient was brought in to you? Does your answer to this depend on when the directive was written? If so, do you think they should have an 'expiry date'? How specific does it need to be?

Courts in the UK have confirmed that a person's advance refusal of treatment should be respected (*Re T (Adult: Refusal of Treatment)* [1992] 4 All ER 649; [1992] WLR 782). This depends, however, on the 'consent' or 'refusal' being valid. Cases have confirmed that an advance directive will be valid, provided it was made:

- by a competent patient . . .
- voluntarily . . .
- on the basis of sufficient information . . .
- and is applicable to the circumstances that have now arisen.

This last requirement can be particularly difficult, but if you decide in good faith that the directive does apply (and you have documented this appropriately), you are advised to honour its terms. This common law position is retained and clarified by the Mental Capacity Act 2005 (see below).

✿ What do you think should be required to ensure that consent is valid?

Consent

To be considered valid, consent should be voluntary, informed, continuing and made by a competent individual. There is a case law ruling that consent given by a patient who may have been coerced or under duress to make a certain decision is *not* valid (*Re T (Adult: Refusal of Treatment)* [1992] 4 All ER 649; [1992] WLR 782).

Consent is considered to be 'informed' when the patient has received relevant information necessary to make a decision. Interestingly, the law requires doctors to give as much information as a reasonable doctor would provide; in contrast, the GMC requires doctors to give such information as would be required by a 'reasonable patient'. Such information includes details of common side-effects and risks, as well as information on the potential benefits and the consequences of both treatment and non-treatment.

✿ How much do you think you ought to tell someone about a procedure to ensure that they give informed consent? Think about this in relation to:

- taking blood
- taking a chest X-ray
- performing an endoscopy/bronchoscopy
- performing a vasectomy.

Types of consent

Consent can be verbal or written, and it can be explicit or implied. In other words, if somebody rolls up their sleeve and holds their arm out when you ask to take a blood sample, this is implied consent, which is just as good as them saying, 'I give consent for you to take my blood'. Note that a signed consent form does not *prove* that a patient gave informed consent, it only *proves* that they signed their name on the form. Therefore, when obtaining a patient's consent, the goal is *not* to get the form signed but to ensure the patient gives informed consent. Although in theory verbal consent can be valid for any procedure from venepuncture to an anterior resection, in practice, you will usually need to get the form signed, following the Department of Health's introduction of standardised consent forms.

Capacity for consent

The law is pretty clear that a person's valid consent or refusal of treatment should be respected. However, to give 'valid' consent, a person must have 'capacity', or 'competence' to make decisions.

✿ What do you consider to be important factors in determining a patient's competence to give consent?

✿ Who should obtain consent for which procedures?

British courts considered this matter in a case about a man suffering from schizophrenia, who was an inpatient at Broadmoor Prison Hospital (*Re C*

(Adult: Refusal of Treatment) [1994] 1 All ER 819; [1994] 1 WLR 290; [1994] 1 FLR 31; [1994] 15 BMLR 77). The man, C, developed gangrene in two of his toes. His consultant surgeon believed that he required a below-knee amputation to save his life. The surgeon felt that C's chances of survival without amputation were about 15%, but C stated that he would prefer to die with two feet than live with one. The courts considered whether the mental illness sufficiently reduced C's capacity to understand the nature, purpose and effect of the proposed amputation, therefore making his refusal invalid. The test described by the High Court in determining an adult's capacity to give consent was as follows.

✱ Can the patient:

■ take in and retain treatment information?
■ believe the information?
■ weigh that information, balancing risks and needs?

The judge decided that, despite his mental illness, C was able to do all of the above, therefore making his refusal of consent valid. In the absence of treatment, C's gangrenous toes fell off by themselves and his health was not otherwise affected.

Subsequently another case of (*Re MB (Adult: Medical Treatment)* [1997] 8 Med LR 217 at 224) clarified the test, but it did not include the criterion of belief. The need to believe information is not incorporated into the test of capacity in the Mental Capacity Act 2005 either, which is expected to come into force in 2007. It is worth remembering that, as a doctor you play a role in assessing someone's capacity. The language you use, the time and place in which the assessment takes place, the opportunity for questions and discussion all have a bearing on whether or not a patient can understand, retain and consider what you are saying.

✿ Considering the '*Re C* test' in the present case, think about whether the patient with motor neurone disease would have been competent to give consent at the time he made his feelings known. We know that the patient in this case had impaired ability to communicate but we are not given any information as to his mental capacity.

✿ This patient's disease was described as 'aggressive and rapidly progressive'. Do you think that time could have been a factor in his emotional state and therefore affected his ability to make a competent decision on his views on resuscitation? Is emotional state relevant to the assessment of capacity using the *Re C* (as amended by *Re MB*) criteria? If so, how?

Prisoners and consent

✿ Do you think prisoners have their autonomous decisions respected? Should they be able to give consent and decide what happens to them, or should this right be removed?

This concept has been tested in English common law (*Freeman v Home Office* [1984] All ER 1035; [1984] 2 WLR). A prisoner serving a life sentence claimed that he was unable to give consent as he felt he could not really refuse treatment recommended by those who have the power to discipline him. The initial ruling affirmed this idea, but the Court of Appeal found that there had been no coercion although it did not need always to consider the facts of the case as to whether consent can be valid before accepting it. For example, if a doctor has the power to influence a patient's situation and decision, that patient's consent may not be valid. This could happen in all cases, not just those involving prisoners.

Prisoners are able to give consent, the same as anybody else. The validity of the consent must, however, be certain before it is acted upon.

'Do not attempt resuscitation' (DNAR) orders

Decisions regarding the 'resuscitation status' of patients in hospitals are essentially advance directives. These should, ideally, be made following discussion together with the patient, but this is often not possible. In cases where the patient is not competent to make a decision, it is the responsibility of the doctor in charge of the patient's care to act in the best interests of the patient. The courts have confirmed that it is good practice to involve relatives and loved ones in decisions relating to the treatment of incompetent adults (*F v West Berkshire Health Authority* [1989] 2 All ER 545, HL).

✿ Sometimes DNAR orders are assigned to competent patients without their knowledge on the basis of 'clinical futility'. Is this right? What happens where you work?

✿ Sometimes DNAR orders are *withheld* from patients in situations even where resuscitation would *not* be in their best interests, simply because their son/daughter is a medical professional or other hospital employee. Should this have any effect on the care that a patient receives? Whose best interests are at stake in such circumstances?

✿ Do you think that relatives should be able to make decisions on the resuscitation status of a patient? Why/why not? Imagine what it would be like to have a relative who is unconscious in hospital. Remember the need for a doctor to consider the patient's best interests and think about the wider situation of the patient's surroundings when you consider their 'best interests'. For example, how does the involvement and wellbeing of the family affect the patient? Will it help the patient to get better if they have strong family support? Are the family necessarily best placed to be the patient's advocate or represent his or her views, even if the family cannot give proxy consent?

✿ Can you imagine a situation where the relatives may not have the best interests of the patient at the forefront of their minds? Although most relatives are good judges of what patients would want, this is not always the case.

Clinicians only have a 'snapshot' of the patient's life and it is dangerous to make assumptions about the quality of the relationship or altruistic motives based solely on familial roles. See Case 3 for more on this.

Quality-of-life issues

It is an important part of any decision that a doctor makes in the 'best interests of the patient' to consider the quality of life that would result from any treatment that is administered. Saving somebody's life is not necessarily what the patient would want, as was demonstrated by the wishes of the man in this case. Putting his competence to make decisions aside, he was evidently thinking that life on an artificial ventilator would not be the kind of life that he would want to live. So often in medicine the philosophy of 'active treatment' means that care providers want to do everything they can to help their patients, and it may be difficult for them to accept that sometimes the best thing to do is nothing. However, some ethicists have argued that the notion of 'prospective autonomy' (the ethical basis for advanced statements) is problematic because the human condition is such that we can rarely know how we would feel in extremis (even if we believe that we do now).

Acts and omissions and the doctrine of 'double effect'

✿ Consider this question: Is the discontinuation of life-saving treatment any different from not initiating the treatment in the first place? If you do think there is a distinction between *withdrawing* and *withholding* treatment, on what basis would you argue the distinction? Does one appear more 'active' than the other? Do you believe the morality is to be found in the act or omission rather than the consequences? Does one seem to be more on a par with euthanasia than the other? If so, why?

The debate of 'stopping' versus 'not starting' is often used to illustrate the arguments that theorists have employed to distinguish between acts and omissions.

In a philosophical 'thought experiment' the issues around this real or imaginary distinction are illustrated by that of two uncles, both with a rich baby nephew from whom they stand to gain the entire inheritance if the nephew dies. Both uncles go up to the bathroom whilst the nephew is having a bath with the intention of drowning the child. The first uncle goes up to the bathroom and does just that. The second uncle goes up to the bathroom but as soon as he wants to drown his nephew, the baby's head slips under the water and the uncle watches him drown. Is there a moral difference between the two uncles?

✪ This example is used by both the supporters and opponents of the Act and Omissions distinction to support their argument. How do you feel about it? Do you think the uncles are both equally guilty of the babies' deaths or do you think the uncle who watched the child die is slightly less culpable than the one who actually pushed him?

Similarly, views about withdrawing treatment differ. Some argue that withdrawing treatment is no different from not starting treatment in the first place, while others believe once treatment has started, withdrawing is equal to euthanasia.

Another related argument is the 'doctrine of double effect'. This is an ethico-legal term (see *R v Cox* [1992] 12 BMLR 38) used in situations where one action may have two possible effects and separates the intention from the outcome. The Doctrine states that an act with a good intention is permissible, even if it has a foreseeable (even inevitable) bad consequence. The Doctrine is consequentialist in nature, in the sense that it suggests the ends justify the means. This is in contrast to Kantian ideology which diametrically opposes the idea.

✪ A thought experiment used to illustrate the Doctrine is the very politically incorrect story of 'Fatty in the Cave'. In the story Fatty and his friends are potholing when Fatty gets stuck in one of the narrow passages and blocks everyone else inside the cave. The other pot-holers have some dynamite which they can use to blast a hole to get them out, even though this has the inevitable consequence of also blowing up Fatty. The Doctrine dictates that this is permissible. Do you agree?

✪ Can you really separate the moral value of an act from its foreseen effects, or are they intrinsically linked?

73

✿ Can you think of any other applications of the Doctrine of Double Effect in moral discussion? How might the Doctrine be used to strengthen Bush and Blair's case for war in Iraq?

The one medical application of the Doctrine of Double Effect is when morphine is used to relieve pain in terminal care. The doses prescribed may also have the side effect of depressing the respiratory system and hastening death.

The intention is beneficent, ie to alleviate pain with effective analgesia, but there might be a foreseen 'double effect'. Some people feel that, as long as the intention is to treat pain and not to kill, this is acceptable. However, there are those who believe that the intention is not important – it is the outcome (death) that matters, and that may be a good thing or a bad thing. Similarly, views about withdrawing treatment differ. Some argue that withdrawing treatment is no different from not starting treatment in the first place, whereas others believe that once treatment has started, withdrawing it is equal to euthanasia.

✿ Thinking about withdrawing treatment – what do you consider to be 'treatment' and what do you think is a basic requirement of life? Are the following treatments or are they fundamental to life?

- Antibiotics to treat infection (where the primary diagnosis is cancer)
- Intravenous fluids
- Tube feeding.

Issues surrounding the withdrawal of treatment are discussed in detail in the case of Tony Bland, a football supporter who was left in a persistent vegetative state following the Hillsborough Disaster in 1989. The case was eventually passed to the House of Lords (*Airedale NHS Trust v Bland* [1993] 1 All ER 521; AC). In this case, Lord Goff stated that where a patient lacks capacity, a treatment can be discontinued where its use is no longer considered to be in the patient's best interests. Although doctors and medical students rarely need to read entire legal judgments, the judgment of Lord Goff of Chieveley in the *Bland* case is very important, as it provides a detailed analysis of the ethics and law surrounding this difficult and complicated issue. The case of Tony Bland now has to be read in the light of an on going case involving a man called Leslie Burke, which is discussed opposite.

The difficulty for the doctor lies in assessing the best interests of the incompetent patient, and it is important to remain alert to how your own values and beliefs about the sanctity of life and quality of life will influence this determination. New guidance from the GMC[1] is a useful reference, and, of course, the patient may have made an advance statement, which describes what he or she would perceive to be in his or her 'best interests' in the event of incapacity. Indeed, the greater use of advance statements and the use of patient proxies to represent the incapacitated patient is a cornerstone of the legislative changes in the Mental Capacity Act 2005. It will be interesting to see whether these statutory developments make the assessment of an incapacitated patient's best interests any less vexed and complex.

However, should the patient be competent to make decisions for themselves, they would be able to say whether they wanted the treatment to continue. It is unusual, though not impossible, for a patient who is receiving artificial ventilation to be conscious and legally competent to decide on the future use of the ventilator. One situation where this could feasibly occur is in the case of motor neurone disease, where patients may be of sound mind. In such cases, the patient may be able to pull the endotracheal/tracheostomy tube out, therefore removing their own treatment. Other patients may be unable to move enough to do that. They could well be capable of deciding that they do not want the ventilator, but they would need help in the physical action of removing the equipment.

Therefore, if you thought that this patient's advance directive was valid in the first instance, you may consider it right to stop the ventilation. Or, if he turned out to regain consciousness and capacity after the arrest incident, he may ask you to remove the tube. If you were the doctor in charge and you considered that the advance directive was invalid but that continuation of artificial ventilation was no longer in the man's best interests, you may decide to remove the treatment. In summary, there is no right answer to this dilemma; as elsewhere you need to be able to apply ethical principles to the context of the particular situation.

The cases of Diane Pretty and Leslie Burke

The high-profile case of a 43-year-old woman with motor neurone disease may have crossed your mind when discussing the above situation (*R (on the application of Pretty) v Director of Public Prosecutions* [2002] FLR 268). It may be worth considering that in this woman's case she was not asking for any treatment to be removed. She said that she wanted to commit suicide and because she was unable to perform the act of putting pills in her mouth and swallowing them, or performing any other act of suicide, she asked the courts to allow her husband to help her do what she would otherwise do by herself. The House of Lords ruled that, despite the patient's competence and autonomy, she was asking for her husband to perform an act of assisted suicide, which is not legal in the UK. The Human Rights Act 1998 did not affect the previous law, and the court essentially ruled that it was most important to protect life (under article 2, the right to life) and protect the vulnerable (those disabled people who might feel pressurised to accept assisted suicide). See Case 25 for more information on the Human Rights Act.

✿ Do you agree with the House of Lords' ruling in the case of Diane Pretty? Or would you have allowed her husband to help her to die?

✿ Diane Pretty took her case to the European Court of Human Rights where she ultimately lost her battle. Why do you think this was?

Ironically, the verdict was delivered just a few hours before the UK High Court granted another 43-year-old woman, known as 'Miss B', the right to die. (Re B (Adult: Refusal of Medical Treatment) [2002] 2 All ER 449). The crucial difference between the two cases was that Miss B was asking for a treatment to be stopped (a ventilator switched off), whereas Diane Pretty was requesting an intervention to help her to die.

✿ Is there an ethical difference between these two actions if the intention and the outcome are the same?

Diane Pretty died in May 2002, two weeks after the ruling and after 10 days of pain and breathing difficulties. She said of the court decisions: 'The law has taken all my rights away.'

Conversely, the recent case of Leslie Burke concerns a man who has cerebellar ataxia, a degenerative brain condition, which will eventually lead to loss of speech and movement; he will require treatment by way of artificial nutrition and hydration to keep him alive. Mr Burke was afraid that when he became unable to communicate, although he may still be conscious of what was happening to him, artificial feeding would be withdrawn with the effect that he would be starved to death. He therefore wishes to create an advance directive that will ensure hydration and nutrition continues, even if doctors believe that life-prolonging treatment is no longer in his best interests. Mr Burke sought judicial review of the GMC guidance (Burke v the General Medical Council [2004] EWHC 1879) on withholding and withdrawing life-sustaining treatment, arguing that doctors should not be able to withhold or withdraw treatment (nutrition and hydration) on the basis of 'quality of life'. On 30 July 2004, Mr Justice Munby ruled in favour of Mr Burke in the High Court. The GMC lodged an appeal on 30 September 2004. At the time of writing, the GMC's appeal had not been heard. Anyone practising, or training to practice medicine should be aware of this case, however it is eventually resolved.

Communication issues within the healthcare team

In this situation the nurse on the ward told the arrest team leader that the patient had signed an advance directive. This raises some important issues about communication and the importance of keeping accurate records of actions in healthcare.

✿ Should it be the responsibility of the nurse looking after a patient to ensure that cardiac arrest teams are not called if the patient suffers an arrest? If you are a doctor on the cardiac arrest team and you are the first to arrive at the scene, should it be up to you to check the patient notes to find out if they are meant to have attempts at resuscitation, or should you start until somebody tells you otherwise?

All NHS trusts will have policies on decision-making regarding resuscitation and communication. Although these policies will be drawn from national guidance (eg the United Kingdom Resuscitation Council (UKRC) and the BMA), there may be local variation and it is important to familiarise yourself with the local guidance and procedures on resuscitation decisions when you begin working in any clinical setting.

Allocation of resources

Resources are always limited in healthcare, and rationing decisions therefore have to be made all the time. A patient who is successfully resuscitated following a cardiac arrest is usually transferred to an intensive care unit (ICU) for further treatment. Beds in ICUs are always in short supply, as well as presenting a huge cost to the health service.

✿ If a patient does not wish to be resuscitated in the event that they suffer a cardiac arrest, should the limited resources and funding influence the decision about whether or not to respect their wishes? Furthermore, if you think that it is acceptable to include resource constraints in the moral analysis of whether or not a patient should be resuscitated, who should have responsibility for weighing the claims of competing groups to, and allocation of, scarce resources?

Summary

■ In UK law, a competent person's advance refusal of treatment should be respected.

■ **Valid** consent is voluntary, informed, continuing and made by a competent individual.

■ Capacity to give consent is specific to individual decisions, and should be assessed using the legal test established in the case of *Re C* and revised in *Re MB*.

■ In England and Wales, people may not appoint a legal power of healthcare attorney to make proxy decisions. They may soon be able to do so under the new Mental Capacity Bill.

■ In situations where patients are not competent to give consent, doctors may treat if it is in the best interests of the patient, having regard for the patient's medical and other (eg spiritual, cultural, familial) interests.

Reading

- BBC. www.bbc.co.uk/religion/ethics/euthanasia/
- British Medical Association. www.bma.org.uk – go to ethics, then physician-assisted suicide.
- Chan SY. Whose life is it anyway. *BMJ* 2005; 330: 486.
- Martin DK, Emanuel LL, Singer PA. Planning for the end of life. *Lancet* 2000; 356: 1672.
- Voluntary Euthanasia Society. www.ves.org.uk
- GMC, Seeking patients' consent: the ethical considerations, Nov 1998 (www.gmc.org/standards/consent/htm).
- *Case of Pretty v United Kingdom.* See the European Court of Human Rights website (www.echr.coe.int and search HUDOC for Application no. 2346/02).

Reference

1. General Medical Council. *Withholding and Withdrawing Life-Prolonging Treatments.* London: GMC, 2002.

CASE 3: THE INCOMPETENT ADULT AND ADVANCE DIRECTIVES

Issues

Advance directives
Relatives
Proxy consent and the Mental Capacity Act 2005
Adults with Incapacity Act (Scotland) 2000
The law on euthanasia in the Netherlands – recent developments

Sue is a 56-year-old solicitor. She becomes aware that her memory is deteriorating rapidly and her grasp of what is going on around her is loosening. She is diagnosed as having early-onset Alzheimer's disease. While at this stage, she completes an advance directive in consultation with her GP, a family friend.

Nine months later, the disease has progressed rapidly, to the extent that Sue no longer recognises her immediate family. Following a bout of 'flu, she is admitted to hospital with suspected pneumonia. Her husband, Donald says she should not be given an antibiotic, in accordance with her advance directive. He says that this was exactly the situation she had contemplated while still able to express her wishes. Sue's 35-year-old daughter Sally is vigorously insisting that you pull out all the stops and treat her mother as you would any other patient with a respiratory infection.

- **Do you give Sue antibiotics?**
- **What influences your decision?**

Use this page to write down your own ideas

Advance directives

✱ Remember that in the UK an advance refusal of treatment is respected provided that the initial directive was valid.

✿ How can you be sure that Sue's advance directive relates to this specific situation? Even if you are satisfied that the advance directive is sufficiently specific to be an expression of Sue's wishes in the event of developing pneumonia, how can you be sure that it still represents her present views?

Relatives

The views held by a patient's relatives can have a substantial influence over the care that a patient receives. Legally, in England and Wales, relatives have very few rights in determining medical care, but good medical practice recognises that there are in fact several 'parties' in most medical cases. The emotional and psychological effects suffered by relatives who are not kept as informed as they would like, or who perhaps feel that their loved one is not being treated in the way that they would like cannot be over-stated.

Proxy consent and the Mental Capacity Act 2005

The only way that a relative of an adult patient can make official decisions on medical treatment is if they have 'Durable Power of Healthcare Attorney'. Durable Power of Healthcare Attorney can be given to an individual when a patient feels they may not, in the near future, be able to make their own decisions about medical treatment. Once a person has been given this power of attorney in areas where this is given legal recognition, they make decisions as a 'proxy'.

This has not yet achieved legal recognition in England and Wales, although in Scotland adults may appoint a 'proxy decision-maker' and in many parts of the United States legislation has given decisions of people such binding force. A proxy decision-maker is somebody who makes a person's decisions on their behalf. This currently only occurs in England and Wales with medical treatment for *children*, in which case the parent or legal guardian is able to make 'proxy' decisions.

However, the position in relation to adults will change in England, Wales and Northern Ireland once the Mental Capacity Act 2005 comes into force, probably in 2007. Under this Act, adults will be entitled to appoint proxy decision-makers to take treatment (and some non-treatment) decisions on their behalf, in the event of becoming mentally incompetent.

The background principle will remain the 'best interests' test, although this will now be more clearly laid out in a checklist. The reforms will also lead to the creation of a new Court of Protection, which would monitor proxy's decisions and also appoint managers to oversee some cases.

It therefore is – and will remain – the doctor's duty to act in accordance with the wishes and best interests of the patient. If this includes going against the wishes of the patient's loved ones, attempts may be made to discuss the issue with the relatives with the aim of reaching a mutual agreement.

✿ How might you discuss the issue with Sue's daughter?

✿ Would you explain that you are treating Sue according to her own wishes?

✿ Would you tell the daughter that it is not uncommon for patients who are very unwell not to receive antibiotics? Antibiotics are potent drugs with many side-effects. If these side-effects cause substantial discomfort (eg diarrhoea) and outweigh any potential benefits, they may not be considered appropriate.

✿ What else would you like to discuss? Is there anything you would not want to talk about?

The Adults with Incapacity Act (Scotland) 2000

✿ What do you think about relatives giving consent on behalf of adult patients? What are the potential benefits of this? Can you imagine any possible problems that may arise?

The Adults with Incapacity Act (Scotland) made it legal to give or withhold consent on behalf of other incapacitated adults in Scotland. The Act covers affairs relating to the property, finances and welfare of 'incapable adults'. The welfare part of the Act, which relates to medical treatment, came into force in 2002. Under the Act, 'incapacity' is defined as being:

- incapable of acting; or
- making decisions; or
- communicating, understanding or remembering decisions.

This could be due to a mental disorder or an inability to communicate due to physical disability. Most people protected by the Act will have a form of dementia or learning disability or will have suffered an accident or head injury. Capacity is task-specific: some patients may be capable to give consent to intravenous hydration but unable to give consent for a coronary angioplasty, because the procedure is more complicated.

When faced with an adult who lacks capacity, healthcare workers must make efforts to contact the person who has been designated their welfare attorney/guardian. This is most likely to be the next of kin. The public guardian can be contacted if it is unclear whether the patient has a welfare attorney/guardian, or if you do not have their contact details.

As a doctor you must make treatment decisions through consultation with the patient's welfare attorney. They should have full access to information, as any *patient* would, so the GMC has changed its guidance regarding breaching confidentiality in this respect. When you treat an incompetent adult you must aim to:

- benefit the adult
- only provide treatment that provides benefit
- choose the least restrictive option
- take into account the past and present wishes and feelings of the adult
- consider the views of relevant others.

If the welfare attorney disagrees with the doctor regarding treatment, a second medical opinion should be sought. If there is still disagreement the matter can be taken to court for resolution.

In order to treat an incompetent adult, the healthcare professional should complete a form (S47), which details why the adult is incompetent in this case and the treatment plan proposed. This can be done in the absence of a welfare attorney if the patient does not have one, but it must be completed. The form is valid for the duration of the treatment plan, up to a maximum of 12 months. Note that this Act does not cover emergency treatment. If an incompetent adult requires immediate treatment to save their life or safeguard their health, this can be administered without delay. For more information, visit the BMA website (www.bma-org.uk).

The law on euthanasia in the Netherlands – recent developments

An explicit policy on euthanasia began to develop in the Netherlands in the early 1970s. At first purely jurisprudential, this policy was officially legalised in 2001. Despite much international attention, this legislation was largely symbolic and practice remained relatively unchanged.

The most important discussions currently taking place in the Netherlands are about the qualifying conditions for euthanasia, which have always formed the very core of the policy. These so-called 'due care' criteria stipulate that a doctor can only be exempt from prosecution for euthanasia if he or she is satisfied, among other things, that the patient has made a voluntary and well-considered request and that the suffering is unbearable and without prospect of improvement or relief. The act of euthanasia must therefore be both autonomous and beneficent. This is interesting because it goes directly to the heart of one of the most important debates in bioethics, namely whether autonomy is pre-eminent in the 'four principles' model (see Chapter 4). Furthermore, if autonomy is pre-eminent, pain and suffering is a subjective question: beneficence can only be determined by the individual patient. However, if there has to be some objective determination of pain and suffering, then this suggests that beneficence and autonomy are equally weighted in the context of the Dutch law.

Recently, however, two cases in particular have highlighted situations in which there appears to be a conflict between these two principles. In the 1994 *Chabot* case (Chabot BE, *Zelf beschmikt*.utig.Balans) the Supreme Court ruled that psychiatric suffering might qualify for euthanasia under the 'due care' criteria. The court wanted to limit the suffering to the psychiatric rather than psychological suffering so as not to *appear* to de-medicalise the criterion completely. Currently, the *Brongersma* case (2000 and 2001) is causing controversy on the matter of whether or not the 'life fatigue' of very elderly people who are simply 'finished with living' might similarly constitute suffering so unbearable as to qualify for euthanasia under the criteria.

On the one hand, if suffering is to be considered as subjective, if a person wishes to die their pain must almost by definition be such that it is 'unbearable' according to the 'due care' criteria. On the other hand, the implications of the acceptance of non-medical suffering within euthanasia are potentially extremely significant. The medicalisation of all suffering changes notions of 'illness' and, subsequently, the role of the doctor. It might also increase fear of all suffering and that associated with old age in particular. No example better illustrates the potential tension between beneficence and autonomy.

The Brongersma case – a summary

Edward Brongersma was a former senator and prominent public figure who, aged 86, was 'tired of life' and felt that 'death had forgotten him'. He had repeatedly asked his GP, Philip Sutorius, to assist him in his suicide and in April 1998 his request was granted. The public prosecutor consequently instigated criminal proceedings against Sutorius on the grounds that he did not adhere to one of the 'due care' criteria, namely that the suffering should be unbearable and without prospect of relief.

In October 2000 the District Court of Haarlem acquitted Sutorius on the basis of expert testimony on the subjectivity of suffering. The public prosecutor appealed against the verdict. In November 2001, on the basis of the testimony of two experts who had been asked to investigate the case, the Court of Appeal in Amsterdam convicted Sutorius of violating the 'due care' criteria. The court judged that 'life fatigue' is a general social, rather than a specifically medical, problem. It should therefore not be considered under the 'due care' criteria of the euthanasia policy, thereby implicitly judging autonomy to be neither the sole nor pre-eminent moral principle applicable to decisions relating to euthanasia.

Following the Dutch House of Lords decision to prosecute Sutorius, the Royal Dutch Medical Association (KNMG) requested an inquest led by Professor JH Dijkhuis to look at the following questions:[1]

1   Are there inherent boundaries within the due care stipulation which exempt a doctor from prosecution after respecting a euthanasia request with regard to 'life fatigue'?
2   In this light, should there be an amendment to the present guidelines of medical practice in this regard?

With regard to the first question, the committee said that the boundary introduced by the Dutch House of Lords is probably not practicably viable. The committee saw four options in terms of the role of 'life fatigue' within euthanasia regulation:

(a)   limiting the role of the medical profession to exclude it
(b)   extending the role of the medical profession to include it
(c)   extending life-fatigue euthanasia to the responsibility of a multi-disciplinary medical team
(d)   excluding life-fatigue euthanasia from all professional domains.

Of these options, the committee favoured option (b), but advises that the KNMG develop these itself by its continuing engagement with the profession and its role within society. The debate therefore appears to continue . . .

Summary

- Although, legally, a patient's relatives have few rights in medical decision-making, good medical practice requires you to balance relatives' legal rights with the fact that they themselves may need your help and advice.
- New law in Scotland (the Adults with Incapacity Act 2000) makes it possible to make decisions on behalf of other adults.
- Legislative change is proposed for England and Wales which would afford statutory status to advance directives, and encourage adults to appoint proxies in relation to healthcare decision-making.
- Doctors in the Netherlands can be exempt from prosecution for euthanasia if they satisfy strict criteria.

Reading

- British Medical Association. www.bma.org.uk – go to ethics, then physician-assisted suicide.
- Huxtable R. Withholding and withdrawing nutrition/hydration: the continuing (mis)adventures of the law. *Journal of Social Welfare and Family Law* 1999; 21: 339–56.
- www.terrisfight.net – Terri Schiavo's family's campaign; and 'The sad case of Terri Schiavo', *Economist* 23 March 2005. (Two sides of the American version of the end-of-life dilemma.)
- www.livingwill.org.uk

Reference

1. Dijkhuis JH. *In search of norms for the behavior of doctors with requests of life termination in the case of life suffering*. KNMG (Royal Dutch Medical Association), 2004. www.knmg.antsennet.nl Chabot BE, *Zelf beschikt*.Utig.Balans.

CASE 4: THE 15-YEAR-OLD WITH DIABETES

Issues

Duty of care
Competence and age of medical consent

You are an SHO in accident and emergency (A&E). Daniel, a 15-year-old adolescent, is brought to your department by his school friends. They say that he is acting 'weird . . . drunk-like'. They claim that he has not been drinking and does not use drugs; they have spent the afternoon skateboarding in the sunshine. They then depart.

Daniel is brought through to a cubicle and is seen by the triage nurse. His speech is slurred and his movements are uncoordinated. He is aggressive and refuses treatment: 'I just wanna get out of here. . . . Leave me alone you bastards, don't you dare touch me.' While the nurse goes to find you, he runs from the hospital, leaving his school bag behind. You look inside his bag to check for an address, and find vials of insulin and some sugar sachets, as well as his home address.

- **What do you do next?**
- **Do you have a continuing duty of care, now that he has left the hospital?**
- **Whom would you contact? Should you talk to:**
  - **his parents/guardians?**
  - **his school?**
  - **the police?**
- **If he had been 16, would it have made a difference?**

Use this page to write down your own ideas

Duty of care

Hospitals which have no A&E department are not legally obliged to assume a duty of care for patients who turn up on the doorstep. However, the hospital in this case has an A&E department, which means your duty of care started when Daniel entered the hospital; and without proper assessment of the situation you cannot discharge that duty simply because he left the department.

There are several possible explanations for this patient's behaviour:

- He may be hypo- or hyperglycaemic.
- He may be drunk or on drugs, even though his friends have said this is not the case.
- He may have nothing wrong with him at all and just be playing around.

There is a real chance that Daniel may be hypo- or hyperglycaemic. You should suspect this because of the way in which he was brought in and because you found the insulin in his bag. There is therefore the possibility that he may require medical attention and you should make efforts to deliver this.

To try to track him down, there are several options open to you. If you ask the police to help find him, you do not have to divulge anything more about him other than that he needs medical attention. However, it is always best to tell the police your concerns as fully as possible so that they can help in the most appropriate way (eg by not treating him as a dangerous criminal). As part of their search, they will go to his home and contact his parents. The parents may find it more distressing to have the police chasing their son than if they were to hear about the problem through the hospital. For these reasons, it is probably best to contact the parents in the first instance. You will then also be able to build up a fuller history of Daniel that may help to explain his behaviour better.

Bear in mind that when trying to track down patients in this way, you have a duty to respect the patient's confidentiality. However, in this case, you have very little information about Daniel so there is very little you could disclose.

'Good Samaritan' acts

As a doctor you have no *legal* obligation to treat people you meet beyond your medical duties. In contrast with much of Europe, the UK does not have a 'rescuer law', ie a law that requires those with the requisite skill or ability to rescue another person. The only exception is where there is a pre-defined and established duty of care as there is to Daniel when he presents at A&E. This legal duty does not legally extend to doctors outwith the clinical setting. For example, if the captain on an aircraft puts out a call asking if there are any doctors on board, you would not be found negligent in British law if you decided not to volunteer your services (although you may feel a moral duty to assist). However, if you did decide to come forward, you would be offering to assume a duty of care and would be required to perform to the level of your professional capability, and not to that of the general public. You might therefore be vunerable to litigation if things went wrong. It is, however, unlikely that a patient would bring such an action to court, and even more unlikely that a court would find in favour of the claimant. It is in society's interests to encourage skilled people to help in emergency situations without the threat of legal action being a deterrent.

Professionally and ethically, things are different. Some doctors are reluctant to stop at accident sites or offer their services indiscriminately, but most doctors would have a hard time ignoring such a cry for help. In fact, the GMC has stated that there is a *professional* and *moral* duty on doctors to be 'Good Samaritans' if they are sufficiently skilled and have the required expertise. Ultimately, it is still up to the doctor to decide whether they have the skills to be able to help; arguably, a psychiatrist might feel unable to treat a patient injured in an accident.

✿ How would you behave if you came across someone in need of medical attention? Is it ethical to refuse to help? Do you think doctors should be forced to treat in such circumstances?

In some countries, eg France and Germany, doctors *are* required to offer assistance when it is called for. Note that if you are in one of these countries or even on board a Lufthansa or Air France aeroplane, you would also be required to obey the laws of these countries. If you are the sort of person who would offer assistance, make sure you are indemnified by a medical defence organisation that covers 'Good Samaritan acts'.

Competence and the age of medical consent

In the UK, age 16 is the age of medical consent. It is assumed (according to the Family Law Reform Act 1969 in England and Wales; and through common law in Scotland) that people aged 16 or over have the necessary capacity to give valid consent to medical, surgical or dental treatment.

✿ Is age the best measure of competence? Is it ethical?

✿ What happens in cases where a patient has a chronological age of 30 but 'mental age' of 4? (See Case 3.)

If a person **under 16** can demonstrate that they are **competent** to give consent, this can be taken as valid (see Case 2 for more on competence). The legal basis for allowing a minor to consent to treatment in Scotland is established by the Age of Legal Capacity (Scotland) Act 1991. In England and Wales, it is founded in common law as a result of the Gillick case.

The competent minor

The phrase '**Gillick competence**' has become part of common language in the last 20 years, but at the request of the claimant to protect the anonymity of her family, the term has now been formally replaced by '**Fraser competence**' – after Lord Fraser who presided over the case. It is useful to know the background to the case because it has helped to establish the way in which minors are treated in England and Wales.

In 1982, the mother of four girls under the age of 16, was concerned that her daughters may be given contraceptive and abortion advice or treatment without her knowledge or consent. She went to court to try to ensure that this would not be allowed to happen. However, her demands were rejected on this initial trial (*Gillick v West Norfolk and Wisbech AHA* [1984] 1 All ER 365). The judge decided that contraception and abortion advice and treatment are the same as any medical treatment. He decreed that the law must allow competent people under the age of 16 to give valid consent to medical treatment in confidence. It was up to the doctor to decide whether the young person was mature enough to satisfy the conditions of competence.

Mrs Gillick then took her case to the Court of Appeal and won ([1985] 1 All ER 533, CA). The judges overturned the previous decision, stating that parental rights under common law were binding, no matter how mature and independent the young person. Under the age of 16, parents had control over their children and what happened to them, including medical treatment and advice. This implied that doctors could only see or examine a child under 16 with a parent present. The only exception would be in emergency situations, when common law would allow a doctor to treat without waiting for parental consent. The ruling also meant that it became illegal to give information on contraception or abortion to anyone under 16 without parental consent.

The case was ultimately taken to the House of Lords. It was only by a majority of three to two that the Law Lords ruled against the Court of Appeal that parental rights were *necessary* only until a child had reached sufficient intellectual maturity to make their own decisions. Competent people under 16 should be allowed to give valid consent to medical examination and treatment, including that relating to contraception and abortion ([1985] 3 All ER 402). In his ruling, Lord Fraser established the way in which minors under 16 are assessed for competence, often referred to as the '**Fraser criteria**'. A minor can consent to treatment if:

■ they have sufficient understanding of the risks and benefits of treatment/non-treatment
■ they cannot be persuaded to involve their parents, and
■ treatment is in their best interests because their mental or physical health is likely to suffer as a result of non-treatment.

There are certain other things that arose out of this case which have had an impact on medical practice:

■ Under Section 28 of the Sexual Offences Act 1956 (now covered by Section 10 of the Sexual Offences Act 2003) it is an offence to cause or incite a person under 16 to engage in sexual activity. The Law Lords decided that it would not be a criminal offence for a doctor to prescribe contraception for a girl in the best interests of her health. This would not be seen as encouragement if the doctor was sure that without the contraception she would continue to have sex, exposing herself to further risks such as pregnancy, abortion or childbirth.
■ However, as Lord Scarman said: 'Clearly a doctor who gives . . . [a patient] . . . contraceptive advice or treatment not because in his clinical judgement the treatment is medically indicated . . . but with the intention of facilitating her having unlawful sexual intercourse may well be guilty of a criminal offence.' ([1985] 3 All ER 402, 425.) It is not clear where the line is drawn between encouraging sexual intercourse and allowing it.

For further discussion of the *Gillick* case and its issues, go to the law reports referenced in this section or *Medicine, Patients and the Law* by Margaret Brazier (third edition, Penguin, 2003).

In the case of Daniel, from what has happened so far, you cannot assume that he is competent. His mental state may be altered due to an organic cause, eg low blood glucose levels. He may not be aware that he needs to be treated nor of the consequences of refusing treatment. In addition, diabetic teenagers are often in denial about their illness and their need for treatment.

Moreover, there is a legal distinction between consent to, and refusal of, treatment. In the current situation, even a competent refusal of treatment by a minor can be over-ridden (by parents or doctors) until he reaches the age of 18. However, this distinction has been much criticised and seems contrary to the concepts implicit in the *Gillick* case, which establishes competence as the ability to *make* a decision, and does not examine the *content* of the decision. (This is discussed more in Case 5.) In cases such as Daniel's, where a patient aged under 18 lacks the capacity to make a decision, the person(s) with parental responsibility under the Children Act 1989 (usually his parents or guardians) would be able to consent to treatment on his behalf as long as they are seen to be acting in the child's best interests (see Case 11 for more on parental rights).

Summary

- Doctors have a duty of care to people whom they accept as patients.
- Competent patients aged 16 or over can consent to medical treatment.
- The Fraser criteria should be used to assess whether a person under 16 is competent to consent to treatment.
- Parents or guardians of incompetent patients under the age of 18 can consent to treatment on the patient's behalf.

Reading

- Alderson P, Goodey C. Theories of consent. *BMJ* 1998; 317: 1313–15.
- British Medical Association. www.bma.org.uk – go to ethics, and then children.
- Larcher V. The ABC of adolescence; consent, competence and confidentiality. *BMJ* 2005; 330: 353–6.
- *Gillick v West Norfolk and Wisbeach AHA* [1985], 3 All ER 402.

CASE 5: THE 15-YEAR-OLD JEHOVAH'S WITNESS

Issues

Refusing treatment – competent minors
Considering 'best interests'

You are a surgical SHO called to A&E for an emergency standby. Sam, a 15-year-old adolescent, is brought in following a road traffic accident. He had been knocked off his bike, resulting in a complicated fracture of his right femur with major blood loss. He requires urgent surgery.

Sam is lucid on admission and clearly states to you: 'I am a Jehovah's Witness. Please don't transfuse me. Will you promise to contact my church, doctor?' You explain the probable consequences of not transfusing, especially due to the amount of blood he has already lost, and the limitations of artificial blood products. However, he is adamant that he does not wish to be transfused. Shortly after this exchange, he lapses into unconsciousness.

The charge nurse finds an identity card in his wallet confirming that Sam is a Jehovah's Witness, and would refuse a blood transfusion if it were required. The nurses have tried to contact his parents but they have been unable to reach them so far.

- **What should you do next?**
- **May you go ahead and operate, transfusing as necessary, thereby over-riding Sam's express wishes?**
- **Regardless of whether you intend to go ahead and transfuse Sam, should you contact his church as per his request?**

Use this page to write down your own ideas

Refusing treatment – competent minors

It is clear that the law allows competent adult patients the right to refuse treatment (see Case 2). In Case 4 it was explained that competent patients under 16 can give consent to treatment. If we assume that Sam's mental state is normal (and he is not suffering from shock), and that he has made an advance, informed decision to refuse life-saving treatment such as a blood transfusion, then we must accept that he has made a competent decision. So, when a *competent* person under the age of 16 *refuses* treatment, what is the correct course of action?

Competent minors are able to give consent to treatment in the absence of parental consent, and even in the unlikely situation of the parents actively refusing to consent. However, in England and Wales, they are not allowed to refuse to consent, if the parents (or a court) give *their* consent instead. This is virtually saying that the consent of such minors is only valid if it agrees with the medical opinion. As long as either the minor or someone with parental responsibility gives consent, the procedure can go ahead, regardless of the wishes of the other party.

✡ Do you agree with this? Is this an ethically justifiable position? On what grounds?

Considering 'best interests'

✡ What factors do you think are important when determining a patient's best interests? Brainstorm a list yourself before looking at the following paragraph.

The BMA has come up with a list of things that need to be considered[1]:

- The patient's own wishes and values, including any advance statement.
- Clinical judgement about the effectiveness of the proposed treatment, particularly in relation to other options.
- Where there is more than one option, which option is least restrictive of the patient's future choices.
- The likelihood and extent of any degree of improvement in the patient's condition if treatment is provided.
- The views of the parents, if the patient is a child.
- The views of people close to the patient, especially close relatives, partners, carers or proxy decision-makers, about what the patient is likely to see as beneficial.
- Any knowledge of the patient's religious, cultural and other non-medical views that might have an impact on the patient's wishes.

None of these aspects on its own can determine the final decision, and all should be taken into account. The Children Act 1989 and the Children (Scotland) Act 1995 apply specifically to minors and what is in their best interests. The issues at stake in any case include the need to balance the harm caused by violating the young person's wishes with the harm caused by failing to treat. In determining Sam's best interests, it makes perfect sense to contact the church, as Sam has requested, to gather as much information as possible about his beliefs.

However, in situations where time is of the essence, you may not have time to carry out the necessary investigations. If you go ahead and treat Sam you should try to minimise the harm done to him by initially trying alternatives to blood transfusions. There are several alternatives (none as effective as blood), but if they do not work you would have to consider giving him the transfusions.

✿ How would you feel about allowing a competent person under 16 to refuse life-saving treatment?

It is possible that the implementation of the Human Rights Act may force such cases to be dealt with differently in English law – the wish of a competent minor to refuse treatment could be upheld. In Scotland, the situation is also unclear, but it is likely that the decision of a competent minor to refuse life-saving treatment could *not* be over-ridden by their parents or by a court. However, it is doubtful that a court would look harshly on a doctor who acted to save a child's life, even if that meant going against that child's wishes.

Summary

- When a competent patient under 16 refuses consent, doctors can consult with their parents/guardians and the courts if necessary.
- Common law covers emergency situations: doctors can treat patients immediately in situations where it is assumed that consent would be given and if the delay required to obtain consent would cause serious harm to the patient.
- Determining what is appropriate in the best interests of a patient requires consultation with relatives and those involved in the care of the patient.
- Treatment may go ahead if it is in the best interests of the patient but this needs to be carefully considered and 'best interests' does not refer solely to best *medical* interests.

Reading

- British Medical Association. www.bma.org.uk – go to ethics, then children.
- Muramoto O. Bioethical aspects of the recent changes in the policy of refusal of blood by Jehovah's Witnesses. *BMJ* 2001; 322: 37–9.

Reference

1. British Medical Association. *Consent Tool Kit*. London: BMA, 2001.

CASE 6: THE NEGLIGENT SURGEON

Issues

Negligence
Reporting poor clinical practice
Doctors and their families requiring medical treatment

You are an SHO working in A&E. You have noticed that since you started four months ago you have seen several female patients who show signs of sepsis, significant post-operative bleeding and unsightly surgical scars. All of these women have been operated on by Ms Smith, and their complications appear to be a direct result of the surgery. You know Ms Smith well, and she is a very popular surgeon with patients, nurses and doctors alike.

You overhear two theatre sisters discussing how Ms Smith is getting a bit shaky. You suspect that her lack of technical skill is causing harm to her patients – whom you then have to see in A&E to pick up the pieces. Your mother is due to have a hysterectomy in six weeks' time under Ms Smith.

- **Do you tell:**
  - **your educational supervisor in A&E?**
  - **a consultant colleague of Ms Smith in Obs and Gynae?**
  - **your friend, an SHO in Obs and Gynae?**
  - **Ms Smith?**
  - **your mother?**
- **Do you try to make sure your mother's hysterectomy is carried out by another surgeon?**

Use this page to write down your own ideas

Negligence

Among many other things, a doctor can be found negligent due to failure to:

- make a correct diagnosis
- treat
- warn of risks involved in a procedure or treatment.

If a patient believes that a doctor's performance in one of these areas is inadequate, they may initiate claims procedures for negligence. To do this, they must prove that:

- the doctor owed them a duty of care (see Cases 1 and 5)
- the doctor's standard of care was less than should be expected of a reasonable doctor working in that area (a judgment of the court, not of another medic; inexperience is no 'defence')
- the negligence caused them injury which they would not otherwise have sustained and that that injury was reasonably foreseeable, ie not a rare, unpredictable or improbable reaction.

The burden of proof in negligence cases lies with the claimant (ie the patient). This makes it difficult for patients to succeed in negligence claims. Indeed, approximately 70% of cases brought by claimants will fail.

Reporting poor clinical practice

Ever since the Bristol Heart Case[1], where large numbers of operations were performed on children with suboptimal results, legislation and professional codes have been put into place whereby poor clinical practice can (and should) be reported without the person who 'blows the whistle' being reprimanded.

Since the 'Whistle Blowing Act' was passed (see Case 19), the Government has created a structure for 'clinical governance', through which NHS trusts and employees regulate their progress and continuously audit and evaluate their success to improve practice where necessary. As a direct result of clinical governance, individuals are no longer necessarily held personally responsible when something goes wrong. Instead, the hospital will look at what happened and why, and make changes to ensure that the same mistake is not made a second time.

Furthermore, the GMC states in *Good Medical Practice*[2] that patient safety must come first and that all doctors have a professional obligation to report a colleague whose performance puts patients at risk.

Doctors and their families requiring medical treatment

✿ Should the action that you take regarding your concerns about Ms Smith be influenced by the fact that you know your mother is due to be operated on next week?

✿ If you wish to prevent your mother from being operated on by Ms Smith, wouldn't it be ethical to prevent other women from the same fate? Some doctors refer to this logic as the 'granny test': if you would not like your grandmother to be treated in a particular way or by a particular person, no one else should be subjected to it either. This 'test' could just as easily be called the 'father', 'daughter' or 'best friend' test, depending on the circumstances.

Patient demands

In the NHS, no patient has the right to demand that a particular doctor undertakes his or her treatment (although patients do have the right to expect a suitably qualified doctor to explain the procedure to them, so that their consent is appropriately well informed). Equally, patients do not generally have the right to demand treatment and so cannot expect that demand to be met, although they may have recourse to the courts (eg under the Human Rights Act 1998) if they are unfairly denied treatment.

Summary

- Negligence can be due to any failure of care in the chain of investigation, management and follow-up of a patient.
- Negligence claims can be difficult for patients to win, as the burden of proving that the doctor was negligent lies with the patient.
- A successful negligence claim proves that the defendant had a duty of care, that they did not provide the standard of care expected of a reasonable doctor working in that field, and that the injury in question was reasonably foreseeable and occurred as a direct result of the negligence.

Reading

- Brahams D. Impact of European human rights law. *Lancet* 2000; 356: 1433–4.
- Irwin S, Fazanc C, Allfrey R. *Medical Negligence Litigation: A Practitioner's Guide.* Legal Action Group. London, 1995.

– Medical Defence Union. www.the-mdu.com – useful case histories as
well as access to advice.

References

1. The Bristol Royal Infirmary Inquiry. www.bristol-inquiry.org.uk
2. General Medical Council. *Good Medical Practice*. London: GMC,
   1998.

CASE 7: THE SICK COLLEAGUE

Issues

Looking after each other – ethics of working in a team
Risks to patients
Stealing from the hospital
Breaking the law

You are an SHO in anaesthetics. Late one night, after a 'heavy' hospital Christmas party, Clare, a highly competent and popular junior surgical colleague (a fellow SHO), tells you that she thinks she is hepatitis C-positive. You have known her since medical school and often work together in theatre.

The next morning, you are sitting in the coffee room when one of the surgical scrub nurses (a friend of yours) approaches and asks, 'Can I have a quiet word?' She is concerned that drugs, particularly diamorphine ampoules, have been going missing from the controlled drugs cupboard in theatre. There is unofficial but widespread suspicion among the ward staff that Clare has been taking them. Nobody has done anything yet because of her popularity.

- **What do you say to the theatre nurse?**
- **What are your responsibilities in this case?**
- **Do you discuss the issue with:**
  - **Clare?**
  - **another SHO friend?**
  - **your educational supervisor?**
  - **Clare's educational supervisor?**
  - **the GMC?**
  - **no one?**

Use this page to write down your own ideas

Looking after each other – ethics of working in a team

The nature of healthcare means that doctors and other healthcare professionals need to work in teams so that they can deliver the best possible care for patients 24 hours a day. It is essential that everyone is able to work effectively within the team so that this goal can be achieved. It is also important that individuals within the team can ask for and receive support and help from each other when necessary. This is an inherent aspect of working together and directly affects the enjoyment of staff and the quality of patient care. Looking after one another's physical and emotional welfare could include matters like getting coffee or snacks for each other during busy periods, and making sure the workload is fair. It may occasionally be necessary to provide extra support in certain situations and this case illustrates such an example.

The NHS is all about putting the patients' needs first but sometimes this causes the welfare of the staff to be neglected. The irony is that the better the staff are looked after (and look after themselves), the better care they will take of the patients. Working in the NHS, and in healthcare in general, means that staff are confronted by many different sources of stress. It may not be as easy as it is in other lines of work to create a happy and healthy working environment, but it is possible. Making time to socialise together outside work is a good way to enhance team spirit.

✪ Team members need to be able to trust and respect one another. Do you automatically trust other members of the team or does it take time for you to regard them as worthy of your trust? Why?

✪ Patients often trust doctors simply because they are doctors. What do you think about this? Is this trust usually justified? If it is, should you also automatically trust other doctors? If you don't, why don't you?

✪ How do you decide whether you can trust someone? Is there anything you can do or say which will help others (colleagues and patients) to see you as a trustworthy person?

✪ Is it necessary to inform on your colleagues' every mistake or problem? What kind of atmosphere would this create within the workplace? Where do we draw the line, ie how bad must the problem be?

You should consider how much risk the mistake poses to the welfare of others (patients or staff) and whether it is a risk that is constantly present, likely to occur again or a one-off incident. Looking after each other means taking action to help each other within the goal of protecting patients. It does not mean 'protecting' each other in such a way that would jeopardise patient care.

In addition to requiring doctors to act when they believe a colleague's performance presents a risk to patients, the GMC offers specific guidance about working with colleagues and encourages the practice of dealing with problems within the team initially. This may mean speaking to the colleague directly, or asking another team member or senior to become involved. Occasionally, it may be necessary to seek help from outside the team, eg the deanery or postgraduate office in the trust (both useful for doctors in training who have a relatively junior position in the medical hierarchy), the clinical governance lead or trust medical director, the National Clinical Assessment Authority, or the GMC.

A colleague who is taking drugs and/or carrying a serious communicable disease may present a risk to patients. You have a moral and professional duty to protect patients from such risks so you must take action. The question is: What type of action? You must decide at what level you think the problem is best handled. Think about the following issues when making your decision.

Risks to patients

Drug abuse

The first question you must ask is whether Clare is abusing drugs and, if you believe she is, does the drug abuse affect her ability to care for patients. If you believe it does, or it could, you must act quickly.

You should make every effort to find out the facts in this situation before you start making assumptions. If you have a close relationship with this person it may be possible for you to discuss the issues with them. Remember that drug users can be so addicted to the drug that it changes their personality, causing them to lie or steal to keep their habit, when normally they would have never done such things. Furthermore, denial is an inherent symptom of many dependence problems. If the colleague is a friend of yours and they are able to discuss their problem with you sensibly, this is a good start. You can help your colleague while protecting patients at the same time. If the colleague acknowledges the risk they are taking with their own health and the health of patients, they should agree to take some time off and get help from one of the many confidential sources that exist to support doctors, such as the BMA Counselling Service or the Sick Doctors Trust. If there is a senior person with whom the colleague feels able to discuss the problem, this may help. The employer and/or GMC may ultimately need to be informed, and this is best done by the colleague themselves.

Things become more difficult if the colleague denies the problem or refuses to recognise the risk to patients. This is when a senior member of staff should be involved. If there is no such person around, as in the case of a GP who is working single-handed, it may be necessary to contact the employer, find out who the clinical governance lead is and/or consider contacting the GMC yourself. The GMC has the power to remove doctors from the medical register if it decides they are unfit to practise medicine or pose a risk to patients. Abusing drugs is regarded as 'serious professional misconduct'.

✿ What do you define as a 'drug'? Does it matter what type of drug is being used? Are illegal drugs morally or legally different from legal drugs, such as alcohol? Is there a difference between someone who uses cocaine while off duty and someone who gets drunk while off duty?

✿ Would it be as harmful to turn up to work with a hangover from the previous night?

✿ Is your ability to care for patients affected if you have not slept enough or are too tired?

A recent court case (*GNER v Hart; Hart v Secretary of State for Transport* [2003] EWHC 2450 (Civil proceedings arising out of the Little Heck/Selby train crash) where a tired driver was convicted of manslaughter and sent to prison. He had fallen asleep at the wheel and accidentally drove onto a railway track. He caused multiple deaths when a train crashed into his car, and he was convicted on ten counts of causing death by dangerous driving and sentenced to five years in prison. It is possible that a doctor could be found negligent for making a mistake because he was tired. The hours junior doctors work is a hot issue in the context of the European Working Time Directive. In conjunction with the *GNER v Hart* ruling, this means that the chief executive of a trust could go to jail if a doctor was found to be negligent while forced to work outside the EWTD. It is interesting to note that article 4 of the Human Rights Act 1998 prohibits 'slavery' and this provision might even extend to prohibit unfair working times and conditions.

✹ Note that *any* mistake by a doctor, whether or not their ability is diminished by drugs, alcohol or tiredness, may result in the doctor being found negligent in law (see Case 6).

Even if you believe the colleague does not present a risk to patients, you may still want to discuss things with them. Perhaps there is an underlying reason for their behaviour, such as depression. Be aware that the medical profession has a high incidence of depression, suicide and divorce. How would you feel if a colleague committed suicide? By helping to create a climate of mutual care within the team you can also be confident of the support of your colleagues should you ever need it yourself.

✿ What do you think about people who use drugs?

✿ How do you treat patients who you know are drug abusers? How should you treat them?

✿ Do you feel a patient with endocarditis who is an intravenous drug user has less right to treatment than a patient who developed the disease following a dental procedure?

✿ What is your reaction to patients who have contracted HIV infection through a blood transfusion compared with those who caught it through unprotected sex?

✿ How do you feel about smokers and their right to treatment? Do you feel they have less right to healthcare than non-smokers because they played a part in causing their health problems? Perhaps you think they have more right to treatment because they pay more towards their health insurance or to the NHS through tax on their tobacco. If so, are you saying that healthcare should be delivered according to how much you pay for it, not on how badly you need it?

✿ What do you think about people who do other risky activities, eg rock climbing or skiing? What about the self-employed worker who has a myocardial infarction due to a stressful job?

The GMC states that doctors must 'not deny or delay investigation or treatment' of a patient who may have contributed to their condition through their actions or lifestyle.[1]

Serious communicable diseases

The GMC defines a serious communicable disease as 'one that may be transmitted between humans and which may result in death or serious illness'.[1] Examples include HIV, tuberculosis, and hepatitis B and C.

■ Patients

Of course, universal precautions should be used with all patients but how can you further reduce the risks to yourself and others if you know a patient has such a disease? Think about infection control measures such as double-gloving, never re-sheathing needles, wearing a mask, and using 'high-risk' stickers for specimens.

✿ Would you be happy to perform an elective operation on someone who was HIV-positive? If you would be reluctant to do so, would you agree to perform emergency surgery if you were on-call?

If you are exposed to infectious material but do not know whether the patient is carrying a disease, you can try to gain the patient's consent to test them. If the patient refuses, or is unable, to give consent, (eg if they are unconscious) things become difficult. The GMC advice[1] is that in 'exceptional circumstances' you may test a blood sample that has already been taken, but you may not take a new blood sample expressly to test for the disease. Consult your occupational health consultant and be sure you know your hospital protocol on what to do if you are exposed to infectious material.

✿ Do you think all patients should be tested for HIV or other communicable diseases? Why are they not? You may have heard of something that is known as 'HIV exceptionalism', which describes the special processes applicable to testing for HIV. Why might HIV exceptionalism exist? Do you think it should be treated differently? Why?

■ Doctors

Doctors have special obligations regarding serious communicable diseases. The GMC[1] states that if you believe a doctor has such a disease and 'is practising, or has practised, in a way which places patients at risk', the occupational health consultant must be informed or, if necessary, the GMC. Of course, it is best if the infected colleague passes on the information themselves.

Doctors with serious communicable diseases are not prevented from practising medicine altogether. Work activities will only be restricted so that patients are not placed at risk, eg such doctors may not carry out invasive procedures. Medical students, however, are not permitted to register with the GMC if they are known to be infected, although there are moves by the Council of the Heads of Medical Schools to seek refinement of this blanket rule. Furthermore, the Disability Discrimination Act 1995 requires medical schools to consider how they can produce competent house officers by making 'reasonable adjustments' to training.

✿ What do you think medical schools and the GMC should consider in determining how to train students, not just with communicable diseases but with all types of disability and impairment?

✿ Should all doctors be tested for serious communicable diseases? If the GMC has a strict policy on this, why is testing of all doctors not enforced? On what ethical grounds could you reason each side of this argument?

✿ The GMC[1] advises that you should not withhold any investigation or treatment of a patient because they are carrying a serious communicable disease. However, doctors who are carriers of such diseases are not allowed to do procedures that may expose their patients to the same risks. Is this fair?

Consider that doctors (whether they are carrying a serious communicable disease or not) do not need to do invasive procedures on others to maintain their own health. Patients on the other hand may need to be treated to survive.

Stealing from the hospital

✿ How do you feel about the fact that the colleague is stealing diamorphine from the hospital? Is stealing from the hospital the same, morally, as stealing from a different source?

✿ Is stealing ever morally excusable? If so, does it depend on the monetary value of the object, ie is stealing a few paracetamol tablets for a headache better than taking a stethoscope? (See Case 17.)

Breaking the law

Since 2002, all NHS employees have been subject to pre-appointment checks. These checks have been introduced by the Government to tighten up patient safety, as a result of various recent cases including that of Dr Harold Shipman who was convicted of the murders of over 200 of his patients (see Case 24 for more on the legacy of Shipman). Doctors must now let their (future) employers know if they have ever:

■ been charged or convicted of a criminal offence in the UK or abroad (excluding parking tickets)
■ received a police caution, final warning or reprimand.

The GMC should also be informed if a doctor is convicted of a crime. Depending upon the offence it could be regarded as serious professional misconduct with the ultimate penalty of being struck off the medical register.

Doctors are exempt from the Rehabilitation of Offenders Act 1974. This means that whereas other members of the public are allowed to withhold information relating to certain criminal offences which occurred many years ago, doctors must declare all such details, no matter how long ago the incident occurred. In addition, doctors must notify their employer if they have ever been investigated for fitness-to-practise issues in the UK or abroad. Finally, those doctors who may have to treat people under 18 years of age are required to state whether they have ever been investigated by the police or been dismissed from any previous employment for reasons of misconduct.

Employers have a duty to respect confidentiality and act according to the Data Protection Act 1998 when carrying out these background checks. Employers are not prevented from employing doctors who declare that they have been in trouble with the law before, but they would probably not employ someone who lied about any past convictions.

✿ Do you agree that background checks should be done on all medical students and doctors? Do you think these checks are an infringement of personal liberties or a necessary precaution?

The GMC should also be informed if a doctor is convicted of a crime. Depending on the offence, it could be regarded as serious professional misconduct with the ultimate penalty of being struck off the medical register.

Summary

- Doctors have a duty to protect patients if they suspect that they themselves or a colleague poses a risk to the welfare of patients, eg is incompetent due to drug abuse or carries a serious communicable disease.
- Doctors must inform their employers and the GMC if they have ever committed certain offences or been investigated for fitness to practise.
- Patients should receive treatment for their condition regardless of how much they might be perceived to have contributed to their ill health.

Reading

- General Medical Council. Helping doctors who are ill: the GMC's health procedures and GMC Problem Doctors and Fitness to Practice Directorate. www.gmc-uk.org/probdocs/illness.htm
- Sick Doctors Trust. www.sick-doctors-trust.co.uk
- www.paimm.net/ – Integral Care Programme for Sick Doctors. A Europe-wide programme followed by the *Lancet*.

Reference

1. General Medical Council. *Serious Communicable Diseases*. London: GMC, 1997.

CASE 8: DEATH OF A CHILD

Issues

Death certificates
Cremation forms
Notifying the coroner
Post-mortem examinations
Holding an inquest

You are an SpR in paediatric A&E when a six-month-old baby is brought in by ambulance in severe cardiovascular shock. The baby has suffered a respiratory arrest and, despite everything the hospital team does for her, she dies a few hours later. You ask the parents if a post-mortem can be performed on their child to help discover why she died. The parents are naturally distraught and are vehemently opposed to their baby 'being cut up by butchers – can't you leave us to bury her in peace?'

- **How do you deal with the situation?**
- **Should you always ask relatives for consent to post-mortems?**
- **Are there different types of post-mortem?**

Use this page to write down your own ideas

Death certificates

Medical practitioners have a statutory duty to issue a Medical Certification of Cause of Death to the registrar of deaths, *if* they attended the patient in their last illness and have seen the body after death. They must be satisfied that they know the cause and time of death and that this is compatible the patient's circumstances. They must state the cause (not the mode) of death, to the best of their knowledge, in the most specific terms possible.

On the certificate, the actual cause of death is divided into Part I and Part II. Part I should be completed with the disease or condition which directly led to death, eg coronary artery disease. The more specific you can be, the better, because mortality statistics will then be more accurate. Part II relates to other significant conditions that contributed to, but were not directly related to, the cause of death, eg diabetes mellitus.

A common mistake is to fill in the certificate with information that would mean the death should be reported to the coroner. Causes such as 'fractured femur', 'alcoholic cirrhosis' or 'drug overdose' will be rejected by the registrar unless the coroner has been notified.

Cremation forms

If a body is to be cremated, as a great proportion of bodies are nowadays, then there is no chance of the body being exhumed if a death later turns out to be suspicious. Therefore, extra precautionary measures are taken (in the guise of more bureaucracy). After you have filled in the first part of the form, containing information similar to that on the death certificate, a second medical practitioner who has been qualified for more than three years (usually a pathologist), fills in the second part, usually after having discussed the case with yourself and one of your colleagues and after having seen the body to corroborate your story.

Do not complete a cremation form until a death certificate has been issued.

✿ Doctors receive money for completing a cremation form, colloquially known as 'ash cash'. What do you think of this payment?

A practical point, but one which also relates to integrity, honesty and ethical practice is that these payments are taxable and the Inland Revenue is aware of their existence.

Notifying the coroner

If there are any doubts about the circumstances of the death, the case should be discussed with the coroner's office (or the procurator fiscal in Scotland). The coroner is legally and sometimes medically qualified and may choose to hold an inquest, with or without a jury. The coroner should particularly be informed about deaths in the following circumstances:[1]

- When the certifying doctor has not seen the patient professionally in the 14 days leading up to the death.
- Where the cause of death remains unknown.
- Where the death occurred after surgery.
- When the cause of death may not have been natural or may be suspicious.
- Where the death may have occurred from industrial disease or poisoning.

It is then up to the coroner or procurator fiscal to decide whether to investigate the death by holding an inquest and/or a post-mortem on the body. The family cannot prevent a post-mortem from going ahead if the coroner/procurator fiscal has requested one to be carried out. It is therefore inappropriate to ask for consent for a post-mortem in these situations. However, it is good practice to inform the family that it may be necessary and why this is likely to be the case.

Post-mortem examinations

Other occasions when a post-mortem may be indicated are when it would be of benefit to research, education or clinical practice. In these situations the family should be consulted and asked to consent.

Ever since it emerged in the 1990s that organs and tissues were being retained by certain hospitals without the consent of relatives, gaining consent to this practice has become a great deal more explicit. Indeed, this principle is enshrined in the Human Tissue Act 2004, which will come into force in 2006. The Act demands 'appropriate consent' (eg, from parents) for non-coronial post-mortems, although post-mortems will still be able to occur without such consent. Standard forms are often used to make sure that all the requirements for consent are fulfilled.

✿ What do you think about how dead bodies should be treated? How do you treat dead bodies, eg during anatomy dissection sessions?

✿ Are you aware of factors that might influence the ways in which a family responds to death and dying, eg cultural and religious factors, local rituals and rites, and media representations of organ donation, post-mortems, etc?

✿ Is it right that relatives can object to a post-mortem even if it may further knowledge and research into diseases and prevent future deaths occurring? Should they also be allowed to object to post-mortems ordered by the coroner, where the sole benefit will be to establish the cause of death of one individual?

✿ Why is it important for relatives to be able to play a role in deciding the fate of another's dead body? In whose interests are we acting by maintaining this role?

✿ Does it make a difference whether a piece of tissue is kept on a slide in a hospital or buried with the rest of the body?

Holding an inquest

An inquest is an inquiry with the intention of providing the registrar of deaths with the information necessary to register the death. Usually the coroner sits alone, but in certain situations when the death is particularly violent or of public interest then a jury may sit. In this event it is the jury, rather that the coroner who issues the verdict by a majority vote. If you are ever called to give evidence at an inquest, remember that it is an inquiry to find facts and not faults – speak honestly and confidently.

Summary

- If you are unsure about the cause of death, speak to a senior before completing the death certificate.
- Do not complete a cremation form until the death certificate has been issued.
- If the death is notified to the coroner/procurator fiscal, the next of kin should be informed that a post-mortem may be necessary – relatives cannot prevent it from taking place. Consent is superfluous but providing a considered and sympathetic explanation is good practice.
- If a post-mortem is desired for other reasons (eg education or research), relatives must first give their consent and be given accurate information about exactly what will happen to all parts of the body, including organs and tissues. There are standard forms to effect the consent process.

Reading

- The Shipman Inquiry. www.the-shipman-inquiry.org.uk
- Smith G. Dealing with deaths. *BMJ Careers Focus* 2002; 325: 107.

Reference

1. Smith G. Dealing with deaths. *BMJ Careers Focus* 2002; 325: 107.

CASE 9: ORGAN DONATION

Issues

Organ donation and transplantation
Respecting cultural and religious beliefs
Reform of the lasw relating to organ donation

You are an SpR in A&E when a previously fit and well 21-year-old British Asian woman is admitted following a fall from a horse. Her Glasgow Coma Scale (GCS) score is 10 on admission, but steadily worsens and she becomes comatose. You have found an organ donor card in her pocket but when you broach the subject with her parents, they are opposed to this because it is against their religion.

- How do you deal with this?
- Whose wishes should you respect?

Use this page to write down your own ideas

Organ donation and transplantation

After death

Under the Human Tissue Act 1961, people who wish to donate their organs after their death can join an organ donation register and carry a donor card to indicate their wishes. Unfortunately, neither a donor card nor entry on the organ donor register, is binding in law and therefore organ donation does not happen as often or as easily as it should.

In practice, if the relatives are opposed to organ donation it is *their* wishes that are respected more often than those of the deceased.

✿ Why does this happen? How does this compare with the principle that we have already discussed (in Case 2) that no one can consent for another adult?

✿ Is it ethical for us to go against the wishes of someone who wanted their organs to be used after their death?

Currently, a person has no legal right to determine what should happen to their body after their death. It is normally the responsibility of the next of kin, as those 'in lawful possession' of the body, to make decisions as they see appropriate.

The Code of Practice for Organ Transplantation Surgery has been in use since 1979. Its recommendations make clear that before organs are removed, death should be certified by at least two doctors (one of whom must have been qualified for at least five years; neither should be a member of the transplant team, to avoid any potential conflict of interest). The Code confirms that if relatives are against the procedure their wishes should be followed, even if the deceased wished to donate their organs.

The situation for donor organs in the UK is desperate. At present we have an 'opt-in' policy, whereby it is assumed that people do not wish their organs to be used after their death unless they have explicitly requested it. However, if there was an 'opt-out' policy, whereby the situation was reversed and people were effectively required to carry 'non-donor cards', the number of organs available would probably increase substantially. An opt-out system now exists in other countries (eg Austria, Belgium, Denmark, France) although some surgeons are still unwilling to remove organs without the consent of the next of kin.

✿ What are the arguments for maintaining the current opt-in system for organ donation in the UK rather than an opt-out policy?

Live organ donation

✿ People are allowed to donate blood and semen while they are alive. Is there any difference between this and donating a kidney?

The Human Organ and Transplant Act 1989 allows live organ donation to occur between people who are 'genetically related' (grandparents and grandchildren are *excluded*). If a person wishes to be a live organ donor for a 'genetically unrelated person', the Unrelated Live Transplant Regulatory Authority (ULTRA) must first approve the case. ULTRA scrutinises applications to see whether there is any question of payment or coercion, and assesses the motives of the potential donor. Under ULTRA regulations, incompetent persons (adult or child) cannot be live donors because they are regarded as incapable of sufficient understanding to give explicit informed consent.

✿ ULTRA does not currently allow purely 'altruistic' donations, ie donations from strangers. There has to be a pre-existing relationship (marriage, friendship, etc) between the parties. Do you think altruistic donations should be permitted?

The GMC gives specific advice on this issue which reinforces the principles of the Human Organ and Transplant Act.[1] The Human Organ and Transplant Act 1989 makes it illegal for any 'organ' to be bought or sold, whether the donor is alive or dead. Presumably, ULTRA was created to protect donors from coercion. However, although perhaps a *financial* incentive would not exist between genetically related people, there is surely an element of *emotional* coercion that could exist between family members, eg a brother may be put under pressure from his relatives to donate a kidney to his sister. Under the Act, an 'organ' is defined as 'any part of a human body consisting of structured arrangement of tissues which, if wholly removed, cannot be replaced by the human body' and so blood and bone marrow are exempt from the Act.

The live donation of gametes (semen and ova) is covered by the Human Fertilisation and Embryology Act 1990 and regulated by the Human Fertilisation and Embryology Authority (HFEA). Under the Act, it is prohibited for live donors to be paid for their gametes unless it has been approved by HFEA. In practice, sperm donors are paid routinely, whereas egg donors are rarely offered any financial incentive – yet carry the higher risk.

✿ Should sperm and egg donors be paid equally? Is there a problem with paying donors for their gametes? In France, sperm donors are not paid, and they are usually mature men who have already proved that they are capable of fathering a child. Despite this, there seems to be no shortage of willing donors so, at least in France, supply is not a problem.

✿ In some countries organs can be bought and sold on the black market. It is most often poor people who decide to sell a kidney of their own so that they can gain a substantial sum of money. Do you think this is ethical? They are undoubtedly taking a risk with their own health by doing this, and if their other kidney failed at some time in the future, their health would suffer and they could die. It is therefore perhaps not in someone's best interests to lose a kidney. However, the vendor may judge that the health risk is worth taking because their quality of life (with money but without a kidney) may be significantly better than if they retained both kidneys but had no money. Furthermore, other people, such as boxers and racing car drivers, take substantial risks (to health and life) to earn a living, and they are not prevented from doing so. In fact, this risk is usually recognised, and they are financially rewarded accordingly. Do you see any problems with paying donors for their organs? On what ethical grounds could you argue sides of this debate?

✿ Technology is advancing in such a way that it may soon be possible to grow organs in vitro, for transplantation. Do you think this is ethical?

Respecting cultural and religious beliefs

What we regard as 'ethical' is influenced by our cultural, religious, social and family background, as well as our own personal experiences and the legal position of the country in which we live. It is therefore very difficult to argue that one person's set of ethics is more 'ethical' than another's. This is known in bioethics as 'cultural relativism', ie the morality of an act is different, depending on geographical and temporal factors.

In the present day, when many people live within a multicultural society it has become necessary to develop an awareness and a tolerance of different cultural beliefs and customs.

✿ Do you agree that individuals have a right to maintain the beliefs and traditions of their culture or their religion? Are there circumstances when this should not be permitted?

✿ Where do you draw the line between respecting someone's different cultural beliefs and condoning immoral acts? What do you think about circumcisions performed on religious grounds rather than out of medical necessity (male or female)?

In this case the deceased wished her organs to be donated while her relatives refused. It does not matter that they refused on religious grounds they could well have refused because they 'didn't like the idea'. At the current time, the relatives' decision must be respected since the deceased has no right to decide what should happen to the body after death.

✿ Do you agree with this?

It is, however, assumed that the relatives will respect the wishes of the deceased on how the body is treated after death. It should be recommended that people who want their organs to be donated after their death make their wishes known to their family. By initiating discussions on the subject and explaining their beliefs they may be able to encourage the relatives to carry out their request, even if it goes against the personal desires of the family.

Reform of the law relating to organ donation

The Human Tissue Act 2004 is expected to come into force in 2006. This new Act, which is intended as a response to perceived scandals relating to the retention of human tissue, will replace the old Human Tissue Act, as well as the Human Organ Transplants Act 1989, the Anatomy Act 1984 and the Corneal Tissue Act 1986.

The new Act preserves and clarifies much of the existing law. For example, there will remain a prohibition on organ sales, and the donation system will still require a donor to 'opt-in'. The Act is firmly grounded in the notion that consent is a fundamental pre-requisite for the use and retention of human tissue.

However, in the new scheme, unlike under the current law, relatives of a deceased donor will *not* be able to override any consent to donation that the donor gave prior to their death. If the deceased did not indicate their wishes in advance, doctors may still be able to obtain consent from a nominated representative or from someone in a relevant qualifying relationship – the Act lists a hierarchy of individuals who may qualify. The position relating to incompetent adults has yet to be clarified, although it seems likely that the doctor will be asked to consider whether donation can be said to be in that person's 'best interests'.

For our scenario, this seems to mean that the patient's views should be honoured ie donation may occur, regardless of her parents' opposition. However, we would strongly advise awaiting further guidance on how this Act will operate in practice.

125

Summary

- Religion, culture, family, the law and personal attitudes all contribute to forming an individual's set of values or ethics.
- People can indicate how they would like to donate their organs after their death by joining the donor register and carrying a donor card. This is not a legally binding agreement and the relatives should be consulted before organs are harvested.
- The law is due to change in 2006, once the Human Tissue Act 2004 comes into force.

Reading

- General Medical Council. *Transplantation of Organs From Live Donors.* London: GMC, Nov 1992. www.gmc-uk.org/standards/trnsplant.htm
- Human Fertilisation and Embryology Authority. www.hfea.gov.uk
- Kennedy I, Sells RA, Daar AS, et al. The case for 'presumed consent' in organ donation. *Lancet* 1998; 351: 1650–2.
- NHS UK Transplant. www.uktransplant.org.uk
- Schlitt HJ. Paid non-related living organ donation: horn of plenty or Pandora's box? *Lancet* 2002; 359: 906–7.
- www.dh.gov.uk/Home/fs/en – the Department of Health website – search for further information on the Human Tissue Act 2004.

Reference

1. General Medical Council. *Transplantation of Organs From Live Donors.* London: GMC, Nov 1992.

CASE 10: CONFIDENTIALITY AND DUTY OF CARE

Issues

Consent to investigations
Duty of care
Breaching confidentiality

You are a GP in a rural town. Richard, a 35-year-old patient, presents with a dry cough, having recently returned from a four-month-long business trip to South Africa. On the point of leaving the room, he says, 'By the way, I'm a bit concerned – I slept with a woman while away, and I'm worried I might have picked up something'.

You counsel him before taking blood for an HIV test. He returns a week later and you have to advise him that the results show him to be HIV-positive. He is married with two children, and his wife is also one of your patients. He is very upset when you raise the question of discussing the results with his wife. He says, 'No way! Our marriage is in enough trouble as it is!' The couple are not currently sleeping together, although his wife has noticed that he's been trying to avoid any form of intimacy and wonders why.

He then threatens to sue you for breach of confidentiality if his HIV status becomes known to his wife.

- **Do you try to contact the wife?**
- **To whom is your duty of care?**
- **How can you deal with this situation satisfactorily?**

Use this page to write down your own ideas

Consent to investigations

✦ You should always obtain informed consent from a patient before performing any examination or investigation. Failure to do so constitutes an assault and/or battery.

✿ To ensure that consent for a blood test is fully 'informed', what should the patient know about? Does the information they need for a simple full blood count (FBC) test differ from that for an HIV test?

The different types of consent are discussed in Case 2 and the example of blood taking was used in explaining implied consent. In the case of HIV testing, implied consent is not sufficient as they may think you wish to do a simple blood test and not know that you will be testing their blood for this disease. Explicit consent must be obtained from the patient before an HIV test can be carried out; otherwise you risk being charged with assaulting the patient. This has been mentioned in Case 7 and is known as 'HIV exceptionalism'.

✿ Why do we carry out a series of blood tests, such as FBC, liver function tests, urea and electrolytes, without telling patients all the details of all the tests and why we are doing them? Do you think we should be doing this?

HIV tests are covered in the 'duties of a doctor' guidance issued by the GMC.[1,2] Patients are offered counselling both before and after the test is done. The reasoning behind this is to help people deal with a positive result (and the associated stigma and implications for insurance) and to offer advice on safe sex. It is a reflection of the particular context in which HIV and AIDS became news in the 1980s when the public health campaigns highlighted the stigma and devastating effects of a diagnosis.

✿ In the two decades since that campaign, the status and prognosis of an HIV-positive diagnosis have changed considerably. Should 'HIV exceptionalism' now cease?

Duty of care

As a doctor, you have a duty to care for your patients. In a hospital environment, this duty begins the minute they enter the hospital. In the general practice setting, however, this duty is extended so that anyone registered with the practice is your patient, not just when they come and visit you in your surgery.

✿ What implications are there for the GP as a result of this extended duty of care to the wife? When does your duty stop?

Breaching confidentiality

In general terms, a patient's confidentiality should only be breached in exceptional circumstances. You should be prepared to justify such circumstances to the GMC or a court if necessary (see Case 1).

✿ This patient does not want to inform his wife of his HIV-positive status. Do you think that this patient's wife has a right to know about his HIV status, and would you go so far as to inform her of it against his wishes?

✿ Does this situation meet the *W v Egdell* criteria (see Case 1) of presenting a 'serious risk of physical harm to an identifiable individual or individuals' such as to justify (but not require) a breach of confidentiality on the grounds of 'public interest'?

Richard's initial angry reaction could be due to fear and denial: of illness, his own death, losing his family, infecting his wife. You could offer help and support to Richard by being prepared to act as an intermediary in whatever capacity you can. You could also arrange for him to go for counselling with his wife. Both Richard and his wife are your patients. You want to maintain Richard's trust and respect, but at the same time you need to try to protect his wife from becoming infected. You also need to be able to offer her support if she is already infected.

It may be acceptable to go against a patient's wishes and inform sexual contacts of an infection risk. In such circumstances it is important to inform the patient of your intentions before disclosing the information and explain why you feel a breach of confidentiality is justified. If you think that you may need to breach Richard's confidentiality, you should agree on a deadline so that he knows that if he has not told his wife by a certain time then you will tell her. It is also a good idea in this kind of situation to ask him if he would prefer you to meet his wife alone or with him present.

✿ What would happen if you did not ensure that Richard's wife became aware of his infection and the risks to herself, and she subsequently became infected with HIV?

Technically you could be liable for negligence, as it could be said that you failed in your duty of care to the wife (who is also your patient), allowing her to be exposed to further risk of contracting HIV. This emphasises the need for good documentation; recording what you have done, said, advised or recommended as a doctor.

Summary

■ Valid informed consent should be obtained from patients before commencing any examination, investigation or treatment.

■ Consent from the patient must be sought before discussing a patient's case with third parties.

■ Confidentiality should only be breached in exceptional circumstances (as outlined in Case 1).

Reading

- Chalmers J, Muir R. Patient privacy and confidentiality. *BMJ* 2003; 326: 725–6.
- General Medical Council. *Confidentiality: Protecting and Providing Information.* London: GMC, April 2004. www.gmc-uk.org/standards/confidentiality.htm
- General Medical Council. *Seeking Patients' Consent.* London: GMC, Nov 1998. www.gmc-uk.org/standards/consent.htm
- General Medical Council. *Serious Communicable Diseases.* London: GMC, Oct 1995. www.gmc-uk.org/standards/archive/hiv_and_aids_oct_1995.pdf
- Lachmann PJ. Consent and confidentiality – where are the limits? An introduction. *Journal of Medical Ethics* 2003; 29: 2.
- O'Brien J, Chantler C. Confidentiality and the duties of care. *Journal of Medical Ethics* 2003; 29: 36–40.
- Zinn C. Wife wins case against GPs who did not disclose husband's HIV status. *BMJ* 2003; 326: 1286.

References

1. General Medical Council. *Serious Communicable Diseases.* London: GMC, 1997.
2. General Medical Council. *Seeking Patients' Consent.* London: GMC, 1998.

CASE 11: THE YOUNG MOTHER

Issues

Controversial treatment
Prevention versus treatment
Refusing consent for minors
Relationship of trust

You are a GP registrar. Kylie is one of your patients, and is the 15-year-old mother of a 12-month-old baby, Britney. Kylie lives at home with her parents, who help her to look after Britney.

Britney is due soon for her MMR jab (measles, mumps and rubella immunisation). You discuss this with Kylie when she visits for a routine check-up with her mother and Britney. She is completely adamant that she only wants the single jab, not the triple jab since she has heard horror stories about its side-effects. You say that you understand why she is concerned but state that you feel it is in the child's best interests to have the triple jab. Kylie replies that if you will not provide the single jab she will find another doctor who will. In fact, Kylie would rather Britney not be vaccinated at all – 'none of my friends' kids have any of these diseases' she says, 'they're so rare now, I don't see why Brit should be exposed at all'.

The next day, Kylie's mother phones you to say that she wants her grand-daughter to have the triple jab. She says that if she offers to bring the baby in for the jab, Kylie need never know that the baby received the triple rather than the single dose.

- ■ **Does Kylie have the right to withhold the vaccine from her daughter when you feel this would not be in the child's best interests?**
- ■ **As Kylie is under 16 herself, can she legally consent to treatment on behalf of her daughter?**
- ■ **As Kylie is under 16, her mother can make medical decisions on her behalf if necessary. Does this mean that she should/can make decisions for Britney too?**
- ■ **How can you deal with situations when the parent refuses to consent to treatment which you regard as medically indicated for their child?**
- ■ **What are the legal consequences, if any, of doing as the grandmother suggests, by acting expressly against Kylie's wishes and giving Britney the triple jab?**
- ■ **What are the social costs of individual decisions made by Kylie?**

Use this page to write down your own ideas

Controversial treatments

The general public is often influenced in health matters by the press and television. This can be good because it raises awareness of medical issues in society. However, it may also cause anxiety levels to increase when there is no reason to worry. The MMR vaccine is thought to be safe (or even *safer* than the single measles jab) by most medical practitioners. In February 2005, the Japanese government reported that there had been no decrease in the incidence of autism since it withdrew the MMR vaccine. However, the medical circus that arose when the 'link' between MMR and autism was first highlighted means that this is still a public concern. This is presumably at the heart of Kylie's decision to withhold the vaccine from her daughter.

✿ Is it relevant why Kylie is refusing immunisation, or is it enough to know that she is refusing it?

Prevention versus treatment

The purpose of vaccination is ultimately to prevent children from contracting a potentially dangerous disease (eg measles can render a child blind or deaf, and even lead to death). Vaccinating large numbers of children works because it confers the society with 'herd immunity'. This means that the disease is largely eradicated from the population so that the risk of coming into contact with the disease is very low indeed. Therefore, unvaccinated children within the population also benefit from the herd immunity because they are only at a very low risk of catching the disease anyway as it is not around very much. However, herd immunity only works if a certain percentage of the population have been immunised. If there is a large group of children who are not vaccinated, then the risk increases greatly. This risk is not only increased to unvaccinated children but also to those children who are vaccinated because vaccines can only reduce the chances of getting the disease and do not prevent it completely.

Vaccination is a cheap and effective way of reducing the incidence of certain diseases. It is in society's interests to maintain immunisation programmes for all members of the population at risk. Vaccination is, however, not a medical treatment; it is not a cure for a disease that the child actually has. For this reason, parents have the right to refuse immunisation for their child without recourse.

✿ Do you agree that vaccination is not the same as treatment?

You could say that vaccination is in the same class of intervention as a healthy diet or exercise. All are encouraged as important in preventing disease but none are mandatory. However there are other medical interventions such as warfarinising people who have atrial fibrillation, or using β-blockers to control hypertension, that are usually thought of as treatments to prevent a stroke.

✿ Where do we draw the line between prevention and treatment? And whose choice is it to draw that line? Is prevention better than cure? Does it matter if there is a difference between the two, when both improve health?

Choosing not to vaccinate is perhaps more complicated as it has implications for the health of others, even those who are immunised. An analogy can be seen with smoking. By not smoking you will reduce your risk of getting lung cancer significantly. However, if you are around others who smoke, your risk will increase due to passive smoking. Despite this, the UK has not banned smoking in public buildings (although some countries, such as the USA and Italy have done this). Could you envisage nurseries which only allow vaccinated children? In some areas of the USA, children are not allowed to attend school until they have received certain vaccinations.

✿ Britney will only be safe *non*-vaccinated because other children around her *are* vaccinated and have ensured there is herd immunity. Her reduction of risk from adverse effects of the vaccine come at the expense of the other children who *are* vaccinated. In economic terms these consequences are called 'externalities', and Kylie's actions are known as 'free-riding' in the same way as someone who doesn't pay their train fare or dodges taxes free rides public services at the expense of others who do. Can you argue that vaccination should be enforced in the same way train fares and taxes are enforced? What are the grounds for allowing parents the right to choose?

Fluoridation of the water supply is an example of another public health measure that has been cheap to implement and has helped to significantly reduce the incidence of dental caries (although there are some potential side-effects).

✿ Can you brainstorm a list of other initiatives in the UK that have been used to control our behaviour to improve our health? Some examples include making it illegal to travel without a seat belt in cars and setting minimum ages for buying alcohol and cigarettes. Do you agree with these restrictions on personal liberty? Do you believe these measures have been successful? The Netherlands and Italy have no restrictions on buying alcohol, yet have a lower incidence of alcohol-related diseases. Can you think of any other possible solutions to health problems that could be more effective than legislation, eg education?

Refusing consent for minors

Parental rights

As Britney's mother, Kylie has parental rights and therefore the right to decide to refuse vaccination. The current legal situation means that the mother automatically has parental responsibility for her child once it is born, irrespective of marital status. Formerly, if the parents were not married, the mother was the only parent who had *automatic* parental responsibility and therefore the only one who could consent to treatment. However, since November 2003, and following the introduction of the Adoption and Children Act 2001, unmarried fathers also automatically acquire parental responsibility, to be shared with the mother. However, this law does not apply to children born before November 2003; a formal application by these unmarried fathers is still required to obtain parental responsibility. This applies unless a written agreement can be arranged, whereby the mother agrees that the father can have parental rights or there is a court order to this effect or the father is registered as such on the child's birth certificate.

If the two parents disagree between themselves about whether the treatment should be given or not, it may be necessary to take the matter to the courts. For example, this recently happened where two mothers objected to a range of vaccinations for their children (including the MMR jab), although their estranged partners were willing to consent. The court ruled that it was in the children's best interests to receive the vaccinations (*Re C (A Child) (Immunisation: Parental Rights)* [2003] 2 FLR 1095). Although this provides legal authority to support the idea that unilateral consent (ie the consent of one parent) is sufficient, this may present significant professional and ethical dilemmas for the clinician who does not wish to be seen to 'side' with one parent or another, and seeks to maintain a good therapeutic relationship with all parties.

✿ How far does parental responsibility extend? Do parents always have the right to refuse treatment for their children?

Ward of court

In Kylie's case, we cannot *assume* her to be competent because she is under 16. However, if she can demonstrate that she satisfies the conditions of competence set out in the Fraser criteria (simply refusing vaccination for Britney would not allow us to regard her as incompetent) we should respect her right to choose in this situation.

✿ If Kylie was judged to be incompetent, what would be the effect of barring her from being involved in all decisions regarding the care of Britney?

If Kylie was found to be incompetent, using the Fraser criteria, Britney could either be made a ward of court, or the courts could decide to let another party, eg the grandparents, have parental responsibility. Whatever the situation, it would no doubt be important to involve Kylie in any decision-making regarding Britney. Kylie's understanding would increase with age and experience, and her capacity to consent would evolve until she was able to assume full parental control.

In situations where you feel strongly that the parents' refusal to consent is not in the child's best interests, then it may be best to let the courts decide the matter. In recent times, doctors are being encouraged, even expected, to seek legal authority in the event of disagreement with families about treatment decisions. If this is what happens, an application to make the child a 'ward of court' will follow. If the court assumes wardship of the child, all decisions on the medical treatment of the child will be made by the court, acting in the patient's best interests.

In 1981 there was a case which concerned a child born with Down's syndrome and duodenal atresia. The normal course of action is to perform surgery to relieve the obstruction. The parents, however, decided that they would rather the child died naturally over the course of a few days than live handicapped for several decades – they refused consent to the operation. The surgeons believed the procedure was in the child's best interests and took the case to court. The child was made a ward of court but the judge also refused consent to treatment. The surgeons appealed against this decision and the Court of Appeal (*Re B* [1981] 1 WLR 1421) authorised the operation to go ahead. In his ruling, Lord Justice Templeman recognised that the ultimate decision should be based on the evidence and opinions of both the doctors and the parents. He acknowledged that: 'There may be cases . . . of severe proved damage where the future is so certain and where the life of the child is so bound to be full of pain and suffering' that it would be right to allow the child to die. However, he refused 'to terminate the life of a mongoloid child because she also has an intestinal complaint'.

More recently, the European Court of Human Rights examined a case in which a mother complained of a breach of the right to respect her private and family life (article 8 of the Human Rights Act), owed to both her and her disabled son. In treating her son, doctors had used diamorphine against her wishes and had also placed a DNAR order in his notes without her knowledge. The doctors felt that the boy was dying and should be made comfortable. The mother strongly disagreed (and, it is worth noting, the boy was still alive some ten years after the events contested in the case). The court (*Glass v UK* [2004] 1 FLR 1019) found that there had been a violation of the mother's rights and reminded healthcare professionals of the need to reach a consensus or else seek outside advice, such as from a court. This case can serve as a useful reminder of how ethics, law and good communication should go hand in hand. In the case itself, the relationship had broken down so completely that fist fights had broken out between the doctors and the patient's relatives. In a later case, that of severely disabled baby Charlotte Wyatt her parents fought and lost the case to have their child to be resuscitated in event of an arrest.

✿ What is the effect of courts deciding against the views of the parents? Can you think of any other solutions to this problem? How would you deal with parents who refused to consent to treatment on behalf of their child, even though you believe treatment to be in the best interests of the child?

The courts do not always support parents and judgments have explicitly stated a child's best interests to be more than solely his or her best **medical** interests. Increasingly, doctors are being required to seek the advice and authority of the court where there is disagreement between a person or persons with parental responsibility and clinical teams.

Relationship of trust

✿ What would be the effect of giving Britney the MMR without Kylie knowing?

By going against Kylie's wishes you would risk shattering any relationship you have with her, and put in jeopardy any chance of helping Kylie and Britney in the future. Legally, you risk being found guilty of assault and battery, for carrying out a procedure for which you do not have parental consent. It does not matter that Kylie agreed in principle to an injection (the single measles vaccination) nor does it matter that Britney's health is not damaged by the triple jab. Simply by knowingly injecting a substance which the parent had expressly stated they did not want injected into their child, is enough to warrant legal proceedings.

✿ Professionally, doctors are supposed to foster a relationship of trust with their patients. Why is this important?

The more that patients feel that they can trust their doctor to make good decisions, act in their best interests and be truthful with them, the more likely they will be to seek medical attention when necessary. The patient themselves will probably be more honest too, thereby allowing the doctor to make a more accurate diagnosis and give more appropriate advice. Working together on a management plan will mean that the patient is more likely to comply with medication, therefore increasing the efficiency of the doctor's time and energy. Mutual trust within the doctor–patient relationship benefits both parties.

Summary

- Facilitating and supporting the patient's autonomy by fostering a relationship of trust with a patient is important; it will help the doctor to form a more appropriate management plan and encourage the patient to follow medical advice.
- Parents/guardians have the right to refuse consent for their child to receive certain medical treatments (eg routine vaccinations).
- If doctors feel that the parents/guardians are wrong to refuse consent for their child, they can apply to the courts for permission to treat.
- Administering treatment without consent could be regarded as a crime (battery or assault).

Reading

– Axelrod R, Hamilton WD. The evolution of cooperation. *Science* 1981; 211: 1390–6.
– Clements CJ, Ratzan S. Misled and confused? Telling the public about MMR vaccine safety. *Journal of Medical Ethics* 2003; 29: 22–6.
– Horton R. The lessons of MMR. *Lancet* 2004; 363: 9411.

CASE 12: THE ANOREXIC PATIENT

Issues

Confidentiality
Eating disorders and the Mental Health Act
Assessment and the Mental Health Act
Compulsory treatment and the Mental Health Act
Autonomy and paternalism

Mental Health Act Reform

You are a GP registrar, currently attached to a busy student health practice. Emma is a 19-year-old geography student in her first year at university. She temporarily registered with you soon after the start of term in order to be started on the oral contraceptive pill.

While taking her blood pressure, you noticed that she seemed abnormally thin. Her weight and height indicate that her body mass index (BMI) is below average. You mention this, and she says: 'Yeah, I haven't been eating too well – I don't like the food in Hall.'

Three weeks later you are called to her Hall of Residence by the Warden. She tells you that Emma has not been out of her room for three days, and her friends are all concerned about her. Emma refuses to eat anything, saying she is fine and just wants to be left alone.

- **What do you do now? Should you speak to:**
  - **Emma directly?**
  - **her friends?**
  - **her parents?**
  - **her home GP?**

You decide to talk to Emma in her room. She says, 'Why can't you just leave me alone?' and becomes distressed. You suggest that she should perhaps come into hospital for assessment, but she refuses point-blank.

- **Should you force Emma to be admitted to hospital?**
- **If she is admitted, should you force Emma to eat?**

Use this page to write down your own ideas

Confidentiality

Emma is your patient and, as such, is entitled to the same right to confidentiality as any other patient. It is always preferable to try to speak to the patient in the first instance. This is the best way in which to help you form a diagnosis and management plan. If this fails or further information/ support is required, you can ask the patient's consent to speak to others (eg parents, friends, GP, etc). The best way in which to approach this is by suggesting a joint meeting with the patient and the other individual(s). If the patient refuses this, then you have a duty to respect their wishes. However, considering that you are unlikely to have easy access to Emma's past medical notes (because she is only temporarily registered with you), it would be reasonable for you to contact her home GP if necessary. If she happened to be incompetent, you would be justified in breaching confidentiality in her best interests.

Eating disorders and the Mental Health Act

The Mental Health Act 1983, the Mental Health (Scotland) Act 1984 and the Mental Health (Northern Ireland) Order 1986 provide the statutory legislation dealing with mental illness in the UK. There is little difference between them and, for simplicity, specific reference will be confined to the 1983 Act.

The Mental Health Act Commission (MHAC) (and a similar body in Scotland) regulate and provide direction on the implementation of the Act. Refer to the reading list at the end of this case for up to date guidance on these issues.

In order to decide what action is appropriate in this case, you first have to determine whether Emma can be considered under the Act. Patients covered by the Act must have a '**mental disorder**', of which there are four categories: mental illness, mental impairment, severe mental impairment and psychopathic disorder. The Act does not define 'mental illness'; note that dependence on drugs or alcohol, and sexual deviancy (eg paedophilia) are *not* considered 'mental disorders'.

The latest International Classification of Diseases (ICD-10) suggests that for a definite diagnosis of anorexia nervosa to be made all the following criteria should be met:

■   body weight maintained at least 15% below expected body weight
■   weight loss self-induced by avoidance of fattening foods or by one or more of the following: vomiting; purging; excessive exercise; use of appetite suppressants and/or diuretics

- body image distortion with a fear of obesity
- widespread endocrine disorder involving the hypothalamic/pituitary/ gonadal axis
- if the onset is prepubertal, pubertal events are delayed or arrested.

ICD-10 also refers to the occurrence of depressive or obsessional symptoms and the presence of features of a personality disorder. It is also important to exclude somatic causes of weight loss in young patients, including chronic debilitating diseases, brain tumours and gastrointestinal disorders such as Crohn's disease or a malabsorption syndrome.

Without proper assessment, it is impossible to say whether Emma is suffering from anorexia nervosa but you have reasonable cause to believe that she may be. More acutely, you may be concerned that she has abnormal blood chemistry due to her refusal of food. This may be affecting her ability to make the best choice (her capacity) and may compromise her competence as assessed using the *Re C* criteria discussed earlier in Case 2. Legal cases (*Riverside Health NHS Trust v Fox* [1994] 1 FLR 614 and *B v Croydon HA* [1995] 1 All ER 683) have shown that anorexia nervosa can be described as a 'mental disorder' under the Act. The question you must ask yourself is whether Emma should be admitted. If she does need to be admitted, you must then decide whether it is necessary to resort to the Mental Health Act to achieve this, and which section is most appropriate.

Assessment and the Mental Health Act

It is clear that Emma needs proper assessment before an accurate diagnosis and management plan can be decided. Assuming that she does not require emergency treatment, you have several options open to you. In order of preference, these are summarised below.

Voluntary admission

This is always the ideal solution if possible. It may take careful negotiation and expert communication skills to achieve this and it may be worth requesting the help of a social worker (approved under the Mental Health Act). They will have vital experience and, besides, will play an essential part in sectioning the patient if this becomes necessary. If the patient can be convinced to come into hospital voluntarily, this is a very promising start to treatment. It is important that the patient trusts you as their doctor, so you should not lie to the patient or make promises that you cannot keep. Likewise, to avoid being manipulated, do not make deals about what may or may not happen as a result of the admission.

Involuntary admission

If the patient refuses to come to hospital you could decide that a compulsory admission is *not* necessary. This may help to maintain the doctor–patient relationship that could encourage the patient to voluntarily seek your help at a later stage (see Case 11). However, the Act will allow you to admit the patient **involuntarily** if it is 'in the interests of the patient's own health or safety or with a view to the protection of other persons' and the patient is suffering from a treatable mental disorder within the terms of the Act. In the case of anorexic patients, this could be in the situation where the patient's health was threatened by food refusal.

- **Admission for assessment – section 2**
  - **Purpose**: Assessment.
  - **Applicant**: Nearest relative or a social worker approved under the Act. The applicant must have seen the patient in the past 14 days. The applicant is responsible for taking the patient to hospital (although this can be delegated to others, eg ambulance personnel) and, if necessary, may use force (not excessive) to achieve this.
  - **Recommendation**: Two doctors, one, must be a psychiatrist (approved under the Act) and the other should preferably have 'previous knowledge' of the patient (usually the GP).
  - **Duration**: The admission can last for up to 28 days and it cannot be renewed. If an extension is required, a separate application **for treatment (section 3)** must be made. An appeal by the patient can be made any time within the first 14 days.
- **Emergency admission for assessment – section 4**
  - **Purpose**: Assessment. Admission under this section should really only be as a last resort in emergency circumstances. If it **is** necessary, you should aim to get the patient seen by a suitable doctor as soon as possible so that the admission can be approved under section 2 instead.
  - **Applicant**: Nearest relative or approved social worker. The applicant must have seen the patient in the last 24 hours.
  - **Recommendation**: One doctor, who need not be a psychiatrist but who should ideally have 'previous knowledge' of the patient.
  - **Duration**: 72 hours.

Appeals

Patients are allowed to appeal to a mental health review tribunal (MHRT) to overturn the section order. A tribunal consists of a lawyer, a psychiatrist and a lay person, and has the power to discharge the patient. For their appeal, patients may be given legal aid and can obtain an independent medical opinion.

Compulsory treatment and the Mental Health Act

During your assessment of Emma you may determine that she requires treatment for her anorexia. Under the Act, '**medical treatment**' includes 'nursing and care, habilitation and rehabilitation under medical supervision'. For anorexic patients, treatment could take the form of counselling, psychotherapy and nutritional advice.

The Eating Disorders Association in the UK (www.edauk.com) has some specific advice regarding treatment: 'With illnesses like anorexia or bulimia nervosa, the person must themselves want to get better before help can be really effective. People with eating disorders often have mixed feelings about "giving up" their illness. This is because their eating habits have become a way of coping with their profound emotional problems.' This is important to bear in mind when treating these patients: they may initially not want to get better, but to get better they must *first* want to get better. If Emma requires treatment for her anorexia but is refusing, then it is possible to use the Act (section 3, summarised below) to force her to be admitted to receive treatment. Of course, every effort should be made to convince the patient to receive treatment voluntarily, involuntary treatment is unlikely to be very effective in the long-term.

- **Admission for treatment – section 3**
  - **Purpose**: Treatment.
  - **Applicant**: Nearest relative (NR) or an approved social worker. The nearest relative should at least be consulted and if they object, a court order may be needed. The applicant must have seen the patient in the last 14 days.
  - **Recommendation**: Two doctors (see section 2 Recommendation on page 125).
  - **Duration**: Six months. Renewable for another six months and then for periods of a year at a time. Appeals can be made at any time in the first six months, and then once during each subsequent period of renewal.

However, section 3 of the Act can *only* be used on the grounds that the patient:

(a) is suffering from mental illness, severe mental impairment, psychopathic disorder or mental impairment and his mental disorder is of a nature or degree which makes it appropriate for him to receive treatment in a mental hospital; *and*

(b) in the case of a psychopathic disorder or mental impairment, such treatment is likely to alleviate or prevent a deterioration in his condition; *and*

(c) it is necessary for the health and safety of the patient or of the protection of other persons that he should receive such treatment and it cannot be provided unless he is detained under this section.'

✿ The Act makes explicit that it only covers the measures required to treat the mental disorder of the patient. However, what about other interventions such as 'ancillary acts'? For example, what if the patient is ill, eg with pneumonia, yet is competent and refusing antibiotics?

✿ Anorexic patients may require feeding – is this a treatment of the mental disorder too? Can food be regarded as a medicine?

Under the Act, treatment of physical disorders (eg antibiotics to treat pneumonia) can only be given if it is 'sufficiently connected to the treatment for the patient's mental disorder'.[1] Although food is not normally regarded as a medicine, in Tony Bland's case (*Airedale NHS Trust v Bland* [1993] AC 789; see Case 2), the House of Lords ruled that feeding a patient by artificial means could constitute medical treatment. The courts have also accepted that nasogastric feeding can be a medical process, forming an integral part of the treatment for anorexia nervosa (*Riverside Health NHS Trust v Fox* [1994] 1 FLR 614–22). In this case of a 37-year-old woman suffering from anorexia nervosa, the judge recognised that, 'until there is steady weight gain, no other treatment can be offered for the respondent's mental condition, so I hold that forced feeding if needed will be medical treatment for the mental disorder.'

A similar conclusion was reached in *B v Croydon Health Authority* [1995] 1 All ER 683. This case concerned a woman with a psychopathic disorder. When she was held under section 3 she refused to eat to such an extent that she eventually required tube feeding. She brought an injunction against the hospital preventing tube feeding but the health authority appealed. The Appeal Court ruled that tube feeding could be permitted as a form of treatment because it was a necessary precondition for the treatment of the underlying mental disorder.

Consent to treatment for patients admitted under section 3

Under section 63, consent is *not required* for any treatment of the mental disorder in patients who have been admitted under section 3. However, consent should still be sought. A person who is suffering from a mental disorder is not necessarily incapable of giving consent to treatment.

However, the patient may well be entirely able to understand the proposed treatment and its consequences, yet may reject it on irrational grounds, eg in anorexic patients, fear that the treatment will make them 'fat' and her autonomy may well be compromised. Refer to the reading list for some emotive peronalised accounts.

The MHAC 'accepts that some patients with anorexia nervosa may not have the capacity to give and sustain valid consent or that their capacity to consent may be compromised.'[1] Therefore in such situations, section 63 would allow forced feeding of an anorexic patient (detained under section 3, despite them 'competently' refusing consent.

✱ So long as the intervention is directly or indirectly a form of '**treatment**' for the mental disorder, it is permissible under the Mental Health Act.

✿ However, what about non-essential treatment that cannot possibly be part of the management of the mental disorder (eg a hernia repair, sterilisation)?

We have already seen in Case 2 (*Re C (Adult: Refusal of treatment)* [1994] 1 All ER 819; [1994] 1 WLR 290; [1994] FLR 31, 15 BMLR 77), that a **competent** patient (even if they have a mental disorder) has the right to refuse interventions which have nothing to do with the treatment of their mental disorder.

Incompetent adult patients present a different dilemma. In one case, a 36-year-old woman (*F v West Berkshire Health Authority* [1989] 2 All ER 545, HL) with a 'mental age' of five was a voluntary patient in a psychiatric hospital. During her admission she began a sexual relationship with a male patient at the same hospital. Doctors were concerned that she may become pregnant and thought that this was not a good idea because she would be unable to care for the child. They applied to the courts for permission to sterilise the woman. The case eventually reached the House of Lords where Lord Brandon ruled: '[A] doctor can lawfully operate on, or give other treatment to, adult patients who are incapable, for one reason or another, of consenting to his doing so, provided that the operation or other treatment concerned is in the best interests of the patient.' However, the House of Lords suggested that if the proposed treatment was radical and/or irreversible (eg sterilisation), the doctor should seek the advice of the courts before proceeding.

The term '**best interests**' causes a lot of uneasiness in the courts because it can be a very subjective judgement. Sometimes it is not necessarily only the interests of the patient that are considered, but those of their carers or society at large.

✿ Previously, in the USA, some mentally handicapped people were involuntarily sterilised because it was decided that they were incapable of being parents. Arguably, there are many people who may be unfit to be parents (eg paedophiles, drug addicts, girls under 16 years); would it be right for these people to be denied the opportunity to have children too? In whose interests would we be acting, and is it justified?

Autonomy and paternalism

✿ Some people regard involuntary admissions to be an infringement of human rights. They claim the right to be as thin (or fat) as they wish, and question the validity of the diagnostic labels (eg 'obese') imposed by the medical profession. Do you agree with them? Is it possible to be autonomously anorexic?

✿ Forcing people to be detained or receive treatment against their will 'for their own benefit' is a form of paternalism and is thought to be unethical because it denies people their autonomy. Autonomy (the right to self-rule), however, depends on the person being able to exercise this right in normal circumstances. Could a person with a mental disorder be regarded as being incapable of doing this? Does having a mental disorder mean that it may be impossible for the person to be autonomous, simply by virtue of their condition? If autonomy is impaired, would it be impaired in all circumstances or only in some?

✿ Arguably, treatment of their mental disorder may actually restore a patient's ability to make autonomous decisions. Is a temporary 'unethical' action (sectioning the patient and removing their autonomy) acceptable if the ultimate goal (restoring their autonomy) is 'ethical'? Can you think of any situations where this may be unacceptable (eg killing one person to save the lives of two others)? On what ethical principles could you argue both sides: that a particular action would be ethical, and that it would be unethical?

Mental Health Act reform

Recently a new draft Medical Health Bill for England and Wales was put out to consultation. When in due course this Bill is amended and enacted (becomes law), it will have an impact on guidance for the involuntary detention and treatment of the mentally ill. In the meantime, you can find the consultation documents at the Department of Health website: www.doh.gov.uk (search for 'Mental Health Bill').

The proposed reforms of the Mental Health Act extend the definition of mental health disorders considerably and do not specify exclusions. Therefore a patient could be admitted for 'assessment and treatment' of a personality disorder, even if they are notoriously resistant to treatment. The fear is that these reforms will pave the way for abuse of the Mental Health Act to detain unsavoury personalities when there is no evidence for detention under criminal law. Similarly, under the new reforms, doctors will not have the discretion to discharge patients, but rather this will be up to a tribunal in a way similar to release of prisoners from hospital. Mental health activists fear that the Mental Health Act will be used to curtail the freedom of patients and will violate patients' human rights as specified under the Human Rights Act 1998.

Summary

- Strict criteria must be met and certain procedures must be followed in order for a patient with a mental disorder to be compulsorily detained under the Mental Health Act.
- A patient with a mental disorder may be involuntarily detained for assessment and treatment (without their consent).
- Treatment of anorexic patients is most effective if they voluntarily consent to treatment and all efforts should be made to enable this.
- If a patient detained under section 3 requires physical treatment (eg tube feeding in an anorexic patient), this may be delivered without the patient's consent if it is necessary and if it will ultimately help to improve their mental disorder.

Reading

- Barker A. ABC of mental health: mental health and the law. *BMJ* 1997; 315: 590–2.
- British Medical Association. www.bma.org.uk – go to ethics, then to consent and capacity.
- Bridman AM. Mental incapacity and restraint for treatment: present law and proposals for reform. *Journal of Medical Ethics* 2000; 26: 387–92.
- Consultation documents on the Mental Health Bill www.doh.gov.uk (search for Mental Health Bill).
- Darjee R, Crichton J. New mental health legislation. *BMJ* 2004; 329: 634–5.
- Dyer C. High Court detains girl with anorexia. *BMJ* 1997; 314: 845.

- Eating Disorders Association UK. www.edauk.com
- Guide to understanding the Mental Health Act. www.hyperguide.co.uk

Reference

1. Mental Health Act Commission. *Guidance on the Treatment of Anorexia Nervosa under the Mental Health Act 1983*. Nottingham: Mental Health Act Commission, 1997.

CASE 13: THE SUICIDAL PATIENT

Issues

Suicide
Treatment restrictions under the Mental Health Act
Doctors with mental disorders

You are a GP registrar. Patrick, a 74-year-old patient, who is himself a retired GP, presents to your afternoon surgery.

He has been receiving treatment from you for the past four months, since his wife, Joan, died. His mood does not seem to have improved since the first time you saw him. He tells you that he has been feeling suicidal for the past few days. He says he has already worked out what to do and has taken care of his affairs. He asks you for a repeat prescription of his tricyclic antidepressant.

- **What should you do now? Should you:**
  - **write the prescription as requested?**
  - **discuss voluntary admission to the local psychiatric unit?**
- **What would you do if he refuses admission on this basis?**
- **If involuntarily admitted, what forms of treatment for Patrick could be permissible under the Mental Health Act?**
- **Does the fact that he is a doctor make any difference to how you should manage the situation?**

Use this page to write down your own ideas

Suicide

Someone with the medical history of this patient, who has taken such steps to plan his own death, is arguably at high risk of harming and/or killing themselves. In these circumstances, issuing another repeat prescription for tricyclic antidepressants could be dangerous and potentially negligent, or even criminal. Patrick may have not been taking the drug recently, knowing that if he stored up enough pills he could commit suicide by overdosing on them. A better solution to his request would be to acknowledge that the tricyclic was not working and change his prescription to a different medicine that would be safer in cases of overdose.

The Suicide Act 1961 decriminalised committing, or attempting to commit, suicide. However, it does state that 'a person who aids, abets, counsels or procures the suicide of another or an attempt by another to commit suicide' will be held liable for their actions. A person acting to deliberately kill someone would be guilty of murder; a person causing the death of another by acting recklessly or grossly negligently, without any intention to kill, could be found guilty of manslaughter. It is therefore possible, though unlikely, that a doctor who continued to prescribe a tricyclic antidepressant to a patient such as Patrick could face charges of manslaughter or assisting suicide.

✿ If a person wishes to commit suicide, can it be automatically inferred that they must have a mental illness? Do competent people have a 'right to die'? (See Case 2.)

✿ Notwithstanding that doctors suffer high rates of depression and suicide, given Patrick's situation, it is understandable that he may be depressed. In fact it would probably be regarded as *abnormal* if he was not in low mood and instead euphoric about his current situation. Does this mean that his depression is therefore 'normal' or should it be classed as a 'mental disorder'?

Patrick requires a psychiatric referral and may warrant urgent assessment. Obviously, this is most desirable if done with the patient's consent, and every effort should be made to obtain this. However, if he is unwilling and his condition satisfies the grounds for admission under section 2 (or section 4) of the Mental Health Act, then this is the only option available (see Case 12).

Other MHA sections used to detain persons involuntarily with a mental disorder who pose a risk to themselves or others

If this scenario was not set in a GP surgery but instead the patient was in another location (eg home, hospital ward) there are other sections which are important to know about, which can be implemented if necessary in certain situations. Applicants are not necessary for the following sections.

- **Section 5(2)**
  - **Purpose**: Urgent detention of an inpatient.
  - **Recommendation**: One doctor.
  - **Duration**: 72 hours.
- **Section 5(4)**
  - **Purpose**: Urgent detention of a psychiatric inpatient in the absence of a doctor.
  - **Recommendation**: Registered mental nurse.
  - **Duration**: Six hours.
- **Section 136**
  - **Purpose**: Removal to a place of safety (usually an A&E department).
  - **Recommendation**: Police officer.
  - **Duration**: 72 hours.

If the person is refusing to leave a building (eg their house), a magistrate's warrant can be issued which would allow a police officer to enter the premises to remove the person to a place of safety (**section 135**). This can be done on the condition that the person is suffering from a mental disorder, being ill-treated, neglected, not under proper control or is unable to care for themselves (if living alone).

Treatment restrictions under the Mental Health Act

Assuming that Patrick is accepted as having depression (ie a mental disorder within the terms of the Mental Health Act), and requires but is refusing treatment, he could be detained under section 3 of the Mental Health Act. As has been discussed previously (Case 12), '**medical treatment**' has a relatively broad definition for the purposes of the Act.

✿ Normal therapeutic measures for depression include psychotherapy, antidepressant medications and electro-convulsive therapy (ECT). Is it appropriate to administer these treatments under the Act? Do you have any reservations about carrying out any of these treatments without the patient's consent? Should there be any safeguards regarding involuntary treatment?

Treatment under the Mental Health Act is subject to the limitations imposed by certain sections: 63 (see Case 12), 57, 58 and 62.

Treatment requiring consent AND a second opinion – section 57

Some treatments are regarded to be so potentially hazardous that someone cannot automatically be given them *even if they do consent.* These treatments are:

- Any surgical operation for destroying brain tissue or for destroying the functioning of brain tissue (eg lobotomy).
- The surgical implantation of hormones for the purposes of reducing the male sex drive.

In these cases, three people appointed by the MHAC – one doctor and two others (non-doctors) – have to certify that the person concerned has given valid consent to the procedure.

Section 57 does not only apply to people detained under the Act; it applies to all patients.

Treatment which requires consent OR a second opinion – section 58

The treatments dealt with by this section are:

- Long-term medication for the person's mental disorder – This is defined as over three months (since the first dose) during the patient's current period of detention under the Act. In the first three months the treatment can be given without consent, and without the section 58 requirements being necessary. The section is renewed if the type of medication changes.
- ECT – This is done under general anaesthetic and involves passing an electric current through the patient's brain. This induces a type of seizure, and is thought to be beneficial in certain types of depression and other forms of mental illness.

If the patient gives valid consent to treatment, then this must be documented as is routine. The standards of facilitating consent should, of course, be the same as they would be for any patient in any context. If the patient either refuses consent or is incapable of giving consent, then a doctor appointed by the MHAC is needed to provide a second opinion before treatment can go ahead.

Once treatment has been approved a certificate is issued. Certificates must state the plan of treatment in detail. In the case of medication, the types of medication to be given and a range of doses must be documented; in the case of ECT, the number of treatments should be stated. If the plan of treatment is to be changed, fresh certificates are required first. Healthcare staff must check that any treatment administered is covered by the certificate; if it is not, they may be liable for assault.

The provisions of section 58 do not prevent treatment being given in an emergency, as set out in section 62 below.

Urgent treatment – section 62

Sections 57 and 58 requirements do not apply where emergency treatment is necessary to:

- save the patient's life as long as the treatment is not irreversible
- alleviate serious suffering, so long as the treatment is neither irreversible nor hazardous, or
- prevent the patient from behaving violently or being a danger to themselves or to others, as long as the treatment is neither irreversible nor hazardous, and represents the minimum interference necessary.

Doctors with mental disorders

If a doctor with a psychiatric condition comes to you as your patient they should be accorded the same right to confidentiality as any other patient. However, if you felt they posed a risk to their own patients and they continued to practise against your advice, then you should take action (see Case 7). As Patrick is retired, this is not relevant in this case, but it is important to remain alert to the impact of a patient's illness on his or her employment, whether or not they are medical.

Summary

- Patients judged to be at high risk of suicide may be sectioned under the Mental Health Act.
- Treatment under the Mental Health Act is subject to limitations and may require a second opinion to be sought.
- Emergency treatment may be administered without delay in certain situations.
- Doctors who pose a risk to patients due to their psychiatric condition should be advised to stop practising until they are well enough to return to work.

Reading

- Barker A. ABC of mental health: mental health and the law. *BMJ* 1997; 315: 590–2.
- British Medical Association. www.bma.org.uk – go to ethics, then to consent and capacity.
- General Medical Council. *Helping Doctors Who are Ill*. www.gmc_uk.org/probdocs/illness.htm

CASE 14: ABORTION

Issues

Truth-telling and confidentiality
Conflicting rights
Abortion Act 1967

When does life begin?

You are a GP working in a small rural practice. One day a 25-year-old stockbroker, Hannah, comes to see you because she thinks she may be pregnant. You do a pregnancy test that confirms she is at least three months pregnant. She is distraught and tells you that she has known this for nearly two months already and has finally decided that she wants to have an abortion.

She tells you that despite the fact that she is happily married, she does not want the child because she is not ready for a family. She says that she wants to continue with her career at the moment and does not want children for at least another five years. You suggest that she should discuss the matter with her husband before making such a decision. She says that she could never do that because she knows that he really wants to start a family as soon as possible. She asks you to make a referral for an abortion.

A week later, Hannah's husband, Steve comes to see you because he is worried about his wife. He says that she has recently started being sick in the morning and is very tired and irritable. He asks you if she might be pregnant.

■ **What do you say to him?**
■ **How do you deal with Hannah's request for an abortion?**

Use this page to write down your own ideas

Truth-telling and confidentiality

Steve has asked you a point-blank question: Could his wife be pregnant? Take your time to think before you answer. If Hannah had not come to see you beforehand, based on the history and the situation, you could reasonably assume that she may be pregnant. However, she could also have gastroenteritis or another medical condition. You can say this to Steve initially and observe his reaction. By doing this you are preserving Hannah's right to confidentiality, while maintaining your duty to tell the truth.

If you think quickly enough, however, you can find out some more information before you answer sensibly, even without the benefit of knowing that Hannah is pregnant. You could ask why he thinks she might be pregnant – are they trying to conceive? What method of contraception are they using? How reliable is it and how careful have they been?

Once you have asked an initial question or two, Steve's answers will let you know how he stands on the issue. It would have been useful to pose similar questions to Hannah when she had come to see you. If they are not using contraception effectively there is a high risk that Hannah may become pregnant again, and come to you requesting another abortion. This undesirable situation can be avoided by counselling her (preferably together with Steve) about contraceptive methods. This contraceptive advice should be offered as standard to any woman who has an abortion. If you do not feel able to do this yourself, you should refer the couple to a family planning clinic.

Direct questions from patients are often difficult to deflect successfully but you should try not to feel pressured into responding to such questions without thinking first. One thing you must never do is lie to patients, or to others about patients. If you feel that you cannot answer a question truthfully without betraying a patient's confidence, you can simply say that you cannot discuss patient details with the person and ask them to talk to the patient themselves. This advice of course applies to situations in which you need to maintain confidentiality. See Case 1 for a discussion on situations in which you may want to breach confidentiality.

✿ What do you think about lying? Are there times when it is okay to lie? How do you define a lie? Isn't telling the truth or misleading someone as bad as actually telling a lie? Are 'fibs' or 'white lies' acceptable? Do you think it is okay for you to lie because 'everyone does it'?

✿ Why do people need to swear to tell the 'whole truth and nothing but the truth' in court instead of just saying that they will tell 'the truth'?

✿ How do you feel when you lie? Do you ever regret it later? Is it okay as long as the other person does not find out that you lied to them?

✿ How do you feel when you find out that someone has lied to you? How do you feel about that person? Are you content to be lied to as long as you don't find out?

Conflicting rights

Rights of the fetus

✿ What is your ethical standpoint on abortion? Do you feel that a fetus has a right to be born and that therefore the mother has a duty to give birth to the fetus?

✿ Why do you think the way you do about abortion? Are you influenced by your religious beliefs, your parents' beliefs, your friends' attitudes, your personal experiences, or the legal position of your country?

✿ Are there any situations in which you would consider that it is ethical to allow an abortion?

✿ Are there any situations in which you would consider that it was unethical to allow an abortion?

Abortion Act 1967

This Act (amended in 1990) states that a termination of pregnancy may be legally carried out under any of the following circumstances:

- The pregnancy has not exceeded its 24th week and the continuance of the pregnancy would involve risk, greater than if the pregnancy were terminated, of injury to the physical or mental health of the pregnant woman or any existing children of her family.
- The termination is necessary to prevent grave permanent injury to the physical or mental health of the pregnant woman.
- The continuance of the pregnancy would involve risk to the life of the pregnant woman, greater than if the pregnancy were terminated.
- There is a substantial risk that if the child born it would suffer from such physical or mental abnormalities as to be seriously handicapped.

Two registered medical doctors must be in agreement that the grounds of the Abortion Act are satisfied. Only one registered doctor is sufficient in the rare case where an abortion is 'immediately necessary' to save the woman's life or to prevent her from suffering a 'grave permanent injury' to her physical or mental health.

Abortions must be notified and the doctor needs to fill in a form detailing such matters as the method used to date the pregnancy, the grounds on which the abortion was judged to be legal, the methods of diagnosis if the fetal-handicap provision was used, the method of termination, and any complications that resulted.

✿ Do you agree with the provisions of the Abortion Act 1967?

✿ Do you see any problems in the way the Act is worded? It could be argued that in some situations an abortion could legally take place on the grounds that the fetus is female, if what the parents desire is a boy. Is this ethical?

If you disagree with abortions you can refuse to participate in an abortion under section 4 of the Act, which allows for conscientious objection. However, if the woman's health is at risk of 'grave permanent injury' (physical or mental) or her life is in danger and 'immediate action' is required to abort the fetus, section 4 does not apply. In these circumstances doctors must act to protect the woman's life or health, and conscientious objection is not a defence.

The GMC advises that doctors who are morally against abortions should refer the patient to another doctor who practises in accordance with the Abortion Act. Referring the woman is not regarded as 'participating' in the abortion and therefore doctors cannot refuse to do this, even if they conscientiously object to abortions.

✿ Some doctors will organise abortions for any woman who requests one within the first three months of pregnancy. This practice is defended on the grounds that there are statistics that indicate the woman's health is at greater risk if she continues with the pregnancy than if she has an abortion within the first three months. How do you feel about this?

✿ What would be the effect on healthcare if abortions were illegal? In Ireland (and Northern Ireland) termination of pregnancy is unlawful under the Offences Against the Person Act 1861. The life of the unborn fetus must be preserved even if the mother's physical health may be severely damaged. It is also an offence for doctors in Ireland to supply information to women about abortion facilities outside the country. This situation has caused women who wish to have an abortion to go to desperate lengths to have a termination. Recently, a ship equipped with surgical staff and facilities was anchored near Dublin. Irish women were able to board this ship to have an abortion.

When does life begin?

Abortion is a very complex issue, ethically and legally. Part of the reason for this is that there is no firm agreement on when 'life' begins and therefore when a 'right to life' exists.

Ethically

Ethically fertilisation of the ovum the starting point of life?

✿ Many fertilised ova fail to implant in the womb naturally but we do not go to heroic lengths to preserve these 'lives'. Likewise, even after implantation, up to 40% naturally abort.

Perhaps life begins at a later stage, eg when the primitive streak forms (at 14 days), or when brain activity can be detected (at 10–12 weeks) or when the fetus is capable of being born alive (at approximately 24 weeks but this threshold is reducing with advancing technology) or at the point of birth. Some philosophers argue that a being can only be regarded as having moral rights when it can be called a 'person' ie when it has the capacity to value its own existence. This point in development arguably takes place long after birth has actually occurred. See *The Value of Life* by John Harris[1] for this argument.

✿ Do you believe all beings have a right to life? Are there any qualities which a human being must possess to have this right? That is, what makes it immoral to kill a human but permissible to kill an animal or a plant?

Legally

Legally, pregnancy is divided into three stages, based on time:

■ From conception to implantation – Currently, although no court has been challenged on this issue, the Abortion Act only covers the period from implantation to birth. Therefore, contragestive contraception, such as the 'morning-after pill' and the IUD or 'coil', which primarily act to prevent implantation of the fertilised ovum in the very early stages, are not regarded as methods of abortion. The fact that these methods may also work by dislodging an implanted embryo is overlooked because in the first few days following fertilisation (during which these methods are used) it is impossible to prove whether the embryo has implanted or not. Doctors are therefore allowed to prescribe these as ordinary treatments outside the provisions of the Abortion Act. Nevertheless, there are some doctors who conscientiously object to providing contragestive contraception and some pharmacists who refuse to sell the 'morning-after pill'.

- From implantation to 24 weeks – when abortions may be performed on any of the grounds listed the Abortion Act.
- From 25 weeks to birth – when abortions may be performed only on particular grounds listed in the Abortion Act.

Legally, the mother's right to life will always take precedence over the right to life of the fetus. It is only once the child is born, and therefore no longer a fetus, that it is accorded the same legal right to life as any other human being.

Fathers' rights

The Abortion Act gives no rights to fathers; they cannot force the woman to have an abortion or deny her an abortion against her will. In fact, there is no legal obligation to even consult with fathers to hear their opinion – although this may be morally desirable in some cases. The sole gatekeepers of the Abortion Act are the doctor and the pregnant woman.

In one case in 1978, a husband tried to prevent his wife from having an abortion (*Paton v British Pregnancy Advisory Service* [1979] QB 276). The court refused his request and he took his case to the European Commission on Human Rights. He argued that the Abortion Act infringed his right to family life, and his unborn child's right to life. The Commission dismissed his claim ([1980] 3 EHRR 408) on the grounds that these rights must take second place to the rights of the mother – her health and rights were more important in the circumstances. Subsequent cases involving boyfriends, partners and other parties claiming to have an 'interest' in a pregnancy continuing to term have also failed.

✿ Do you agree that fathers should not have any legal rights over the fetus?

Try this series of questions to explore your views on abortion of pregnancy and the ethical basis for your views

1   Do you have definite views about whether abortion is morally justifiable or not? (If not, please go straight to question 4.)

2   If you do have definite views on whether or not abortion is morally justifiable, please identify which moral concepts you draw on to support your views:
    (a)   A woman's 'right to choose'
    (b)   The 'sanctity' of human life
    (c)   Pregnancy as a 'morally neutral' state
    (d)   A balance of risks and benefits
    (e)   Teachings of religion or faith
    (f)   Other (please state)

3   Using your answer to question 2, consider the questions below, which corresponds to the moral concept(s) in Question 2 a–f on which you justify your views (indicated by letter):
    (a)   Is a women's right to terminations unlimited in number to the extent that it may constitute a form of *ex post facto* contraception?
    (b)   When does 'human life' begin? How do you know? Do you object to other contragestive forms of contraception, eg post-coital hormone treatment or IUDs?
    (c)   How can there be moral equivalence between a choice to end a pregnancy and the potential for human life that exists therein and other choices about health, eg the removal of an appendix or gallbladder?
    (d)   Why is it appropriate for anyone other than the woman involved to weigh risks and benefits? If the outcome is poor, does this make a moral act immoral? Conversely, if the outcome is good, does this make an immoral act moral?
    (e)   Is it morally acceptable to subject others to the beliefs of your religion or faith? If it is, why? If it is not, how do you reconcile your belief in the immorality of abortion with accepting that, for society, abortion is acceptable?
    (f)   What is/are the moral argument(s) on which you base your views on abortion? How would you explain choosing this moral position over those described in a–d?

4   If you do not have definite views on abortion, please consider the following moral concepts that are commonly invoked in the abortion debate and state which you find most convincing and why.
    (a)   All women have a 'right to choose' a termination because of the principles of self-determination and autonomy.
    (b)   An embryo and fetus are living entities and therefore should be afforded protection because of the fundamental 'sanctity' of human life.
    (c)   Pregnancy is a morally neutral state and the choice to end a pregnancy is not morally different from the choice to have an appendix or gallbladder removed.
    (d)   Abortion is morally justifiable because the risk of mental or physical harm to a woman who does not wish to proceed with a pregnancy 'trumps' the harms to an unborn and undeveloped fetus. The needs of a fetus are not equivalent to those of an adult.
    (e)   Religion or faith teachings are clear that all living beings (of which a fetus is clearly one) must be protected and not harmed – abortion is morally unjustified.
          Are there any other common arguments you have heard in the abortion debate? If so, what were they? Were they convincing?

5   Can the difference drawn in the Abortion Act 1967 between terminations performed before 24 weeks' gestation and those performed after 24 weeks' gestation be *morally* justified? If so, on what grounds?

6   Will you, as a clinician, elect to exercise your right of conscientious objection and not participate in terminations as provided for under section 4(1) of the Abortion Act 1967? If so, why? If not, why not?

Summary

- Doctors should never lie to their patients, and should maintain confidentiality when appropriate.
- Abortion in the UK is illegal unless covered by one of the conditions under the Abortion Act.
- Doctors who disagree with abortions on principle must refer the patient to a doctor who practises in accordance with the Abortion Act.
- Fathers have no legal right to decide whether a pregnancy should be aborted or not. However, they should be involved in the decision if the mother wishes.
- There is ethical and legal debate about when 'life' begins.

Reading

- BBC. www.bbc.co.uk/religion/ethics/abortion
- British Medical Association. www.bma.org.uk – go to ethics, then to reproduction issues.
- Hewson B. Reproductive autonomy and the ethics of abortion. *Journal of Medical Ethics* 2001; 27 (suppl 2): ii10–14.

Reference

1. Harris J. *The Value of Life.* London: Routledge, 1985.

CASE 15: SEXUAL ABUSE OF MINORS

Issues

Investigation of allegations
Confidentiality and privacy
Consent from minors
Children Acts

You are a GP registrar in an inner-city practice. During a consultation about another matter, David, a 19-year-old patient of yours, tells you that during an argument with his girlfriend, Sarah (aged 18, also a patient of yours), she told him that her father had sexually abused her when she was younger.

You know the family well. Sarah's mother, Rachel (aged 40), is currently pregnant again with her third child. She saw you recently for an antenatal check in the practice. She told you that after a rocky period at home, things were much better, and that her husband was taking a real interest in the family again. For example, he has been helping their younger daughter Jo (aged 13) with her homework.

- **What do you say to David?**
- **Do you inform the police?**
- **Do you make contact with Rachel, Sarah or Jo?**
- **Do you try to talk to the father?**

Use this page to write down your own ideas

Investigation of allegations

On considering this case, your immediate thoughts may turn to the safety of the younger members of this family. It is important in the first instance, however, to remember the source of this information – it is second-hand (ie not from Sarah herself), and it was disclosed during a time when emotions were probably running high and where details may not have been relayed accurately.

✿ How would you go about investigating your concerns?

If you are concerned by allegations it is important not to get out of your depth. False accusations of child abuse can be destroying to families as well as to individuals. There are specific and well-defined procedures for child protection and it is essential that these are followed for the protection of everyone involved. Therefore, it is vital that you always discuss cases such as this with a senior. It should be your consultant or GP trainer who raises the alarm, not you as a junior member of the team. It is important to be alert to the possibility of abuse and, if you are not specially trained in dealing with victims of suspected child abuse, make sure you know where to seek such specialist help promptly.

Confidentiality and privacy

Doctors have a duty to respect the patient's confidentiality. Investigation of this case will lead to an invasion of privacy. If you considered it necessary to make contact with the family, you would have to give careful thought as to how this could be done without causing offence, which may lead to their refusal to co-operate. There are certain situations in which confidentiality may be breached and information disclosed without the patient's permission (see Case 1).

✿ With the above information, do you think you would be able to disclose the possible information that you have about the family? If so, to whom?

Consent from minors

This topic is covered in detail in Case 4. Under the law in England and Wales, children who are 'Fraser competent' can consent to treatment, but they may have their refusal over-ridden. Those who are not considered to be Fraser competent require parental consent to treatment. In these cases it is still considered good practice to involve the child as far as possible in any decision-making processes.

It is possible for a 13-year-old child, such as Jo to have considerable insight into a situation if they are being abused. They may, however, be too afraid to admit abuse, especially if they have been threatened.

Children Acts

The Children Act 1989 and the Children (Scotland) Act 1995 exist to protect the welfare of children. It outlines parental responsibility and guardianship as well as the mechanisms in place for the care and supervision of children whose welfare is considered to be under threat.

Child protection teams are multidisciplinary teams led by social workers brought in to investigate claims of child abuse. They also include doctors, nurses and police officers. Children who are under surveillance due to alleged or confirmed abuse are put on the 'at risk register'. As a doctor, it is possible for you to contact social services to find out if a child is on the register if you have any concerns. Some A&E departments will automatically do this whenever a child comes in. **Child protection orders** and wardship issues are covered in the Children Act 1989 (see Case 11).

Inherent Jurisdiction gives the High Court the power to look after anyone who is unable to look after themselves. This can take the form of an order (for example a care order, an assessment order or an emergency protection order), or it can involve making the child a **'ward of court'**. This is only used in exceptional circumstances. Once a child has been made a ward of court, no decisions regarding their life can be made without consulting the courts first.

Summary

- The Children Act 1989 and the Children (Scotland) Act 1995 exist to protect the welfare of children.
- Courts today prefer to use child protection orders for specific interventions, rather than making children wards of court.
- Child protection work is sensitive and complex and must be handled procedurally correctly by those with special expertise and experience.

Reading

- British Medical Association. www.bma.org.uk – go to ethics, then to children.
- David TJ. Ethical debate: child sexual abuse. When a doctor's duty to report abuse conflicts with a duty of confidentiality to the victim. *BMJ* 1998; 316: 55.
- Johnson CF. Child sexual abuse. *Lancet* 2004; 364: 462–70.

CASE 16: BONE MARROW TRANSPLANT AND FERTILITY TREATMENT

Issues

Fertility treatment
'Motives' for childbearing
Human Fertilisation and Embryology Act 1990
Embryo selection ('designer babies')
Apocalypse now?
Therapeutic cloning
Resource allocation and rationing

You are a GP registrar. A young couple present this afternoon in your surgery. They have one child, Jamie, four years old, who is suffering from leukaemia.

They have been trying to conceive another child for the past two years. They ask you if you will refer them for in vitro fertilisation (IVF). They are quite open in telling you that their primary reason for wanting another child is to provide a source of likely match bone marrow for Jamie, if he needs it.

You know that your local health authority does offer IVF on the NHS, but that the budget has been cut this year, and there are many couples wanting it.

■ **Do you refer them for IVF?**
■ **Do you say anything to them about their motives for having another child?**

Use this page to write down your own ideas

Fertility treatment

✡ What do you think about fertility treatment in general? Is it a 'need' or a 'want'? Should it be available in a publicly funded service, just like any other intervention, or is it a 'bonus'?

✡ Fertility treatment achieves what would usually happen naturally (ie the fertilisation of an ovum by a sperm) in situations where, for some reason, this does not occur. Do you find it a good thing that science enables us to help couples with difficulty conceiving, or do you hold the opinion that conception is a natural process, and if it does not happen this is part of nature and should not be tampered with? Why?

✡ Do you know anybody who has had a child with the help of fertility treatment? Or were you or a friend born as a result of this? Have you seen couples who have had difficulty conceiving?

✡ Is there a right to have a child? Is there a duty on others to preserve such a right? Or do you think the ability to have children is a privilege?

✡ In this case, the couple already have a child. If you think that there is a right to have children, how many children does this extend to? Do they have a right to be given treatment to conceive another child?

See Case 25 for discussion on the influence of the Human Rights Act on reproductive technology.

'Motives' for childbearing

✡ People have children for different reasons. Do you think that there are 'right' and 'wrong' reasons for wanting to have a child? Would wanting to help one of your existing children be a good reason or a bad reason?

✡ How do you think the existing child would feel knowing their sibling had been born in an attempt to help them? Would they feel privileged that their parents had done everything for them? Would they feel some sense of duty and obligation to the younger sibling? How might they feel if their parents did not have another child? Would they feel that more could have been done, and that they were not really valued by their parents?

✡ What about the proposed child? Would they feel that they were alive simply to provide the 'spare parts'? Or would they believe that they had a very special place in the world, and that they had helped their older sibling in a way that nobody else could? Why should you consider a 'future person' in making moral assessments?

✿ If you think that motives for having children can be right or wrong, do your feelings extend to 'types' of parents? Should children be deserved? Should we stop certain people from having children altogether? For example, do you think that drug abusers should be permitted to have a child? If one became pregnant, should their baby be taken into care at birth? Or should they be forced to have a termination? What about prisoners? Should they be allowed to have children? How do you feel about compulsory sterilisation of prisoners?

✿ There are examples in law of people with severe learning difficulties being sterilised because it was feared that they would not be able to look after a child (*F v West Berkshire Health Authority* [1989] 2 All ER 545) (see Case 12). Is this right?

Human Fertilisation and Embryology Act 1990

In 1984 the UK government commissioned a special committee under leadership of Dame Mary Warnock, to look at the ethics of using human embryos. This included both fertility treatments and the use of embryos in research. The committee recommended that embryos be given special status in law. This was accepted by the government, leading to the introduction of the Human Fertilisation and Embryology Act 1990. The Act of Parliament established the HFEA, the government's advisory body for any issues surrounding embryos. There is a code of practice that describes the ways in which the Act should be applied, in the same way as there is a code of practice relating to the application of the Mental Health Act.

Embryo selection ('designer babies')

There has been a growing interest in the media about using IVF as a means of creating and selecting embryos with certain characteristics. This may be for medical reasons, for example two parents who are both carriers of the cystic fibrosis gene may wish to select an embryo that would not have the disease. The development and refinement of pre-implantation genetic diagnosis (PIGD) techniques have greatly increased the ability to 'choose' embryos, and there is a fear that this selection could lead to a widespread creation of 'designer babies' with specific physical attributes, intelligence and other pre-selected desirable traits.

✿ Do you think PIGD and embryo selection should be permitted? If so, how could embryo selection be regulated, to ensure legal compliance?

It is important to give consideration to the above questions prior to formulating any opinion on the morality (or otherwise) of embryo selection.

✿ How do you view the status of an embryo? Do you think that the status of an embryo changes at different stages of its development?

From a legal point of view, day 14 is the limit beyond which research cannot be undertaken on embryos. At this gestation the 'primitive streak' (the precursor to the brain and central nervous system) develops. Although this has been criticised, on the basis that development of the nervous system is continuous from the time of fertilisation, it provides a convenient 'cut off' in law.

Some common ways in which the meaning of personhood and the status of the embryo have been understood and discussed in the ethical literature:

- Persons are characterised by their rationality or capacity for relationships as opposed to mere sentience.[1,2]
- Embryos have the potential to become a person and should therefore be afforded the status of persons from the moment of fertilisation.[3]
- Personhood is a gradual process of development and accordingly the status afforded to the embryo, fetus and eventually child will increase incrementally from conception through pregnancy until birth.[4]

Clearly, if you conclude that the status of the embryo is morally equivalent to that of a person, it is difficult to make a convincing argument for embryo selection, because it would ignore the Kantian principle that all persons should be an end in themselves, and never merely a means to an end. If you believe that the embryo does not have a status morally equivalent to a person, then you need to decide whether embryo selection can ever be ethically acceptable.

✿ Are there any morally sufficient justifications for embryo selection? If so, what do you think these are?

Many people, both clinicians and lay people, could list a number of conditions that they believe would warrant embryo selection. Such examples of justifications could include muscular dystrophy, Huntington's chorea, haemophilia, fragile X syndrome, thalassaemia and sickle-cell anaemia. However, there is unlikely to be a consensus among even the most experienced scientists and clinicians as to an absolute list of conditions that would justify embryo selection.

✿ What are the implications of finding the gene for homosexuality or other genetic traits on the trend for designer babies?

Some people may argue in favour of PIGD and embryo selection on the basis that it enhances their autonomy, as they would be able to make an informed decision about the future of their unborn child. However, the concept of respecting autonomy does not equate to a right to demand treatment.

✿ How should patient autonomy be respected in the context of PIGD and embryo selection?

All assessments as to whether a particular genetic condition is a sufficient justification for embryo selection should be acknowledged to be value judgements. These are the result of personal assumptions about the condition and the meaning of 'disability' in general. The HFEA recommends that information about clinical conditions and the reality of living with a disability should be available to all patients seeking PIGD. This goes some way to acknowledging the difference between the biomedical understanding of a particular disease and the social reality of how that disease affects an individual. For some people, the experience of having a child with fragile syndrome X may be represented as a lengthy and lonely struggle but for others it may be a rewarding and enriching experience in which they feel consistently supported.

How can these, and other multiple realities, be realistically discussed with potential parents? This is perhaps one of the greatest ethical challenges facing those working in reproductive medicine.

Apocalypse now?

In 2003, Louise Brown, the world's first IVF baby, celebrated her 25th birthday as a happy and healthy woman. Earlier in that same year Dolly, the world's first cloned mammal (a sheep) from an adult cell, died prematurely less than two months after the American-based Clonaid claimed that a girl called Eve was born as the world's first human clone. Although Clonaid's claims are largely discredited and the UK strictly prohibits therapeutic cloning, the debate around reproductive cloning of humans continues.

The ethical objections to reproductive cloning relate both to the effects on the cloned person and those on society. The cloned person's physical health is called into question by Dolly's fate. Although there is no reason to presume that the safety of cloning might not improve in the future, the question remains: At what cost? Psychological health is often cited as being at risk for the cloned person. Yet the cloning of a human body is different from the cloning of a 'person' and these adverse effects are purely speculative.

The other objections to reproductive cloning relate to the adverse effects on society. People popularly fear that the technology of cloning makes society vulnerable to the abuses of tyrants and despots. Do you think this is a valid fear?

✿ Do you think that cloning has the same moral status as entities such as bombs and guns, or do you think they are more morally neutral, like computers and phones, which can be used for both good and bad ends?

The argument against cloning for fear of reducing biodiversity is another contentious argument. It is said that 'playing God' will adversely affect the natural richness and diversity of life based on an evolutionary process. And yet many other scientists claim that natural diversity could be preserved by cloning methods which may protect species which are threatened by other aspects of modern technology.

Therapeutic cloning

The public perception of the difference between therapeutic and reproductive cloning is often underestimated, if it is appreciated at all. Medical professionals should lead the way in directing public opinion by judging all these different technologies on their different ethical merits.

Stem cells have the potential to turn into any tissue and their 'cloning' may be the key to research into cures for a huge range of diseases from diabetes to rare congenital birth defects. The stem cells are usually derived from embryonic tissue: 4–7 day old blastocysts discarded following fertility treatment and occasionally embryos from very early pregnancy termination.

✿ This raises important questions again, regarding the moral status of the embryo and its rights not to be violated. Does involvement in medical research violate its rights in these ways? And how do these rights weigh in relation to the rights of people with diseases yet to be cured?

Adult (non-embryonic) stem cells may be found in a variety of tissues such as bone marrow and also have therapeutic potential, as in the case of a man who grew his new jaw in his back.[5] It is argued by some pro-life activists and scientists that adult stem cells should be used preferentially to embryonic stem cells. Yet there are huge cost implications associated with this and thus more resource allocation problems.

In the UK in February 2004 the House of Lords Select Committee supported the government's position in endorsing the use of public funding for stem cell research under supervision of the Human Fertilisation and Embryology Authority. This is in contrast to the US where federal funding for this research has been cut, although it is still permitted to do the work if it is funded privately.

Resource allocation and rationing

This case raises the issue of resource allocation and rationing. Rationing is a very real dilemma in any service where funds are limited. In this situation the couple already have a child. Do you think that this should exclude them from an expensive treatment that other people with no children may also want to receive? Should their reasons for wanting the second child have any influence on your decision to refer them for a treatment that is in short supply? Consider that if these parents are successful, IVF would have created one life and saved another. Is this therefore a better use of resources than giving IVF to another couple who only wish to create one life?

Summary

- Many emotional and psychological issues are involved when children are born following fertility treatment.
- In the UK, the HFEA regulates all reproductive medicine and assisted fertility services, both private and public.
- With advancing technology, it is now possible for people to select certain embryos for implantation. Selection could be on the basis of medical grounds, or simply due to personal preferences – although it is not currently possible to select embryos for cosmetic reasons.
- In a healthcare system with limited resources, ethical issues surrounding the allocation of funding for fertility treatment are particularly complex.

Reading

– Singer PA. Recent advances: medical ethics. *BMJ* 2000; 321: 282–5.

References

1. Harris J. *The Value of Life*. London: Routledge, 1985.
2. Singer P. *Practical Ethics*, 2nd edn. Cambridge: Cambridge University Press, 1993.
3. Locke J. *Second Treatise on Government*. Oxford: Blackwell, 1966.
4. Dworkin R. *Life's Dominion*. New York: Vintage Books, 1994.
5. Warnke PH, Springer IN, Wiltfang J, et al. Growth and transplantation of a custom vascularised bone graft in a man. *Lancet* 2004; 364: 766–7.

CASE 17: SCARCE RESOURCES

Issues

Rationing
Allocation of resources
Quality-Adjusted Life-Years (QALYs)

You are a psychiatrist and are looking after Barry, a patient with paranoid schizophrenia who has been treated successfully in the community for many years. He takes up contact with you and asks to be admitted as he is afraid he will hurt someone. You assess him and decide that he is not an immediate threat to anyone as long as he continues to take his medication, and that he does not qualify for emergency admission. However, you put him on the waiting list for an elective bed, which the primary care trust assures you will be within seven days.

Funding for psychiatric services is currently being reduced due to the development of a paediatric cardiac surgery unit and this means that a bed does not become available within the recommended time. You see Barry twice weekly as an out-patient and although he seems to be doing well, he keeps asking you about getting a bed declaring his ever-increasing emotional distress. After two weeks without a bed he kills his neighbour and then turns the gun on himself.

- **Who is guilty of the killing?**
  - **The patient who continues to be morally responsible for both taking his medication and, in some sense, for actions committed whilst suffering from a mental illness?**
  - **You as the attending medical practitioner, for failing to ensure access to appropriate care?**
  - **The primary care trust for failing to provide adequate financial support to allow appropriate care to be accessed?**
- **How should resources be allocated?**

Use this page to write down your own ideas

Rationing

Healthcare is an expensive business. The population may never have been so healthy and never lived so long, yet still higher standards of health are sought and strived for, at increasing costs. The fact is that improving healthcare provision is a never-ending quest and requires a bottomless pit of resources, no matter where you live or how rich your government is. In the UK, the NHS was set up following the Beveridge Report with the aim of providing a *comprehensive* healthcare system for *all* citizens. However, there is a limit on resources available within the NHS and rationing is an inevitable consequence. There are two forms of rationing:

- **Explicit** rationing dictates allocation of resources according to protocols and guidance.
- **Implicit** rationing is what has always been going on (eg through waiting lists), and is based more on tradition, circumstance and sometimes prejudice.

The current trend is far more towards explicit rationing. The National Institute for Clinical Excellence (NICE) has been a great instigator of this, sometimes resulting in controversial decisions such as restricting the provision of β-interferon to patients with multiple sclerosis, and restricting access to screening programmes (eg the age at which mammograms are offered).

The other way of dividing up rationing is into micro-rationing and macro-rationing. **Micro-rationing** is done between individuals, often on the basis of habit, age or demographic profile. **Macro-rationing** refers to rationing between different types of resources as in Barry's case when resources were allocated to 'sexy' paediatric surgery rather than to 'unsexy' mental health.

Most societies regard healthcare as an important and fundamental service that should be provided. In the UK, the current generation has grown up with the NHS and the idea that access to healthcare should be based upon need and not the ability to pay. The state funds the health service, with minimal costs borne directly by patients (though indirectly it is paid for by those who can afford to contribute through taxes). This may have helped to establish the notion that people have a 'right' to 'free' healthcare. Perhaps it is also because we feel that an adequate standard of healthcare is so important to people's quality of life that it should be provided to everyone – anything else would be inhumane. It could be argued, however, that the standard of education or even housing that one receives has an even *greater* influence on a person's quality of life. Yet we do not allocate people to schools or houses based on their need rather than ability to pay – children with 'low IQs' are not sent to the best schools, while the most intelligent kids are left to go to the worst ones. Why should healthcare be any different?

✿ Do you think people have a right to free healthcare? If so, can this right ever be forfeited, eg by smoking, drinking alcohol or not exercising? How is your answer reconcilable with the requirement described by the GMC that it is unethical to withhold or otherwise change the treatment a patient receives as a result of his or her 'lifestyle'?

✿ Is it ethical to judge whether certain people have a greater right to healthcare based on their contribution (financial or otherwise) to society or whether they are a 'nice' person?

✿ What do you do when you have two 'nice' people or two worthy types of treatment to choose between?

Some would say that doctors should not be empowered to make such judgments. They would argue that doctors are not necessarily the best people to decide on whether a particular person (or a particular treatment) is worth investing in while another is not. However difficult and unpalatable these decisions are, someone has to make them because not everything that needs to be done can get done. The funding of the NHS and healthcare in general is a subject of constant debate and doctors have considerable power in influencing how such matters are resolved.

A study carried out in 1992[1] looked at the factors influencing which patients were admitted to ICU beds. It is widely assumed that such decisions are made on the basis of clinical suitability and the potential benefit of the treatment. The researchers, however, found that during the three-month period (during which nursing shortages reduced the number of beds available) 'political power [in the institution], medical provincialism [one service pitted against another], and income maximisation overrode medical suitability in the provision of critical care services'.[1]

✿ Would you be happy if a close relative of yours was denied treatment on any of these grounds?

✿ On what basis can rationing be done ethically?

Allocation of resources

Theories of justice

You may feel that in allocating precious resources such as healthcare to individuals within a society, it should be done fairly. However, in what way should people be treated justly and equally? Should everyone be given an equal share, or receive a share according to need, societal contribution, or merit? There are several ethical theories of justice that could be employed. Among them are:

- **Utilitarian** – Striving to achieve the greatest good for the greatest number would favour public health measures, eg vaccination, but deny expensive treatments such as heart surgery and intensive care.
- **Libertarian** – These theories have often influenced government policies on health services in the USA. Under libertarianism, there is no *right* to healthcare, it is a *choice*. If people want healthcare they are allowed to pay for it, as with any other commodity or service: they can choose to buy as little or as much of it as they want. This benefits the rich, healthy individuals within a society but neglects the poor and the very sick. However, such a model is virtually untenable socially and even in the USA there is the safety net of Medicaid (for the poor) and Medicare (for the poor elderly), which are funded by the state and aim to provide a minimum standard of health service for all citizens.
- **Communitarian** – The counter-argument to libertarian ideas, these theories aim to distribute healthcare services according to the needs and goals of the community. How these 'needs' and 'goals' are decided upon is not defined and it would be up to the community, eg through democracy, leaders, informed individuals.
- **Egalitarian** – The main aim of these theories is to ensure that everyone has an equal opportunity to succeed in life. Poor health can reduce a person's ability to achieve their goals, and therefore healthcare is provided to prevent this from happening. Beauchamp and Childress[2] describe it as follows: 'Each member of the society, irrespective of wealth or position, would have equal access to an adequate, although not maximal, level of healthcare – the exact level of access being contingent on available societal resources and public processes of decision-making.'

In practice, the application of some of these theories could discriminate people on the basis of gender, race or age. Old age is sometimes (though not overtly) used in some instances as a reason not to provide certain treatments, eg kidney dialysis.[3]

✿ Do you agree with this? Why do you (dis)agree? Perhaps you feel that it is in society's interests to help the younger individuals because they have longer life expectancies and their lives are potentially more useful than those of older people. However, it could be argued that an older person, having worked and contributed to society for 50 years (and even perhaps fought in a World War), *deserves* at least the same right to healthcare as younger members of the society.

Quality-Adjusted Life-Years (QALYs)

The concept of quality-adjusted life-years (QALYs) is an attempt to reconcile the two goals of quantity and quality of life. The aim is to maximise both through health policies. In 1989 the US state of Oregon made policies regarding the state funding of healthcare primarily on the basis of estimates of net benefits to quality of life. Committees ranked the importance of various aspects of healthcare, and therefore how much money should be spent on each area. Certain types of care, such as that of extremely premature babies, were low on the priority list because there was minimal improvement to their quality of life.

✿ Who can judge the quality of another's life and how much a person *values* being alive? There are people who would hate to live if they lost a leg, yet there are wheelchair-bound people who would value their lives just as much as if they lost both legs. People have different thresholds and value life for different reasons. Is it possible to make ethical judgments about another person's quality of life?

Some philosophers argue that it is impossible to choose between people on any basis. One potential solution is to have a form of lottery to distribute healthcare services.

Summary

- Rationing of healthcare resources is necessary in most societies.
- Management plans and treatment options are affected by economic considerations.
- Doctors have an influence on how decisions and funding policies are made.
- There are different ethical theories on the best way to achieve justice through the rationing process.

Reading

- Cookson R, Dolan P. Principles of justice in health care rationing. *Journal of Medical Ethics* 2000; 26: 323–9.
- Edwards SJL, Kirchin S. Rationing, randomizing and researching in health care provision. *Journal of Medical Ethics* 2002; 28: 20–3.
- Ham C. Retracing the Oregon trail: the experience of rationing and the Oregan health plan. *BMJ* 1998; 316: 1965–1969.
- Harris J. *The Value of Life* (London: Routledge, 1985).
- New B. The rationing agenda in the NHS. *BMJ* 1996; 312: 1593–601.
- Rosen S, Sanne I, Collier A, Simon JL. Hard choices: rationing antiretroviral therapy for HIV/AIDS in Africa. *Lancet* 2005; 365: 354–6.[Q24]
- Welsh S, Deahl MP. Modern psychiatric ethics. *Lancet* 2002; 359: 253–5.

References

1. Marshall MF, Schwenzer KJ, Orsina M, et al. Influence of political power, medical provincialism and economic incentives on the rationing of surgical intensive care unit beds. *Critical Care Medicine* 1992; 20: 387–94.
2. Beauchamp TL, Childress JF. *Principles of Biomedical Ethics*, 5th edn. Oxford University Press, 2001.
3. Wing AJ. Why don't the British treat more patients with kidney failure? *BMJ* 1983; 287: 1157.

187

CASE 18: RELATIONSHIPS WITH PATIENTS

Issues

Personal relationships with patients
Professional responsibilities of medical students

You are a heterosexual female final-year medical student, currently attached to a medical firm. You have got to know John, a 21-year-old patient, over the past fortnight. You clerked him in on admission, know his medical history, and have examined him during the course of this time.

Additionally, you have chatted with him each day, and have taken an interest in his recovery. Today, as he is packing his bag to go home, he gives you a 'thank you' card, and asks 'would you like to go for a drink sometime?'

- John is attractive and you have lots in common. Do you agree to go out on a date with him?
- If 'John' was in fact 'Jane' and she suggested you meet up for a 'friendly' night out, would you go?

Use this page to write down your own ideas

Personal relationships with patients

✿ Would you feel comfortable going on a date with a patient? Do you think this situation is in any way similar to a middle-aged patient inviting you round to dinner at their house 'if you feel like getting away from it all and having some home-cooked food'? If not, would this second situation be acceptable?

The GMC gives guidance in *Good Medical Practice*,[1] stating that, 'In particular, you must not use your professional position to establish or pursue a sexual or improper emotional relationship with a patient or someone close to them.'

✿ What do you think is meant by 'improper emotional relationship'? Do you think that there is any other group of people you come across in your work, other than your patients, with whom it would not be appropriate to go on a date?

✿ What do you understand by the term 'professional boundaries'? Why are boundaries seen as important in a therapeutic relationship? What behaviours might enhance or detract from professional boundaries?

✿ Consider non-sexual relationships, eg how will you interact with representatives from the pharmaceutical industry?

Professional responsibilities of medical students

As a medical student, the GMC expects you to adopt the same professional standards as doctors and structures the curriculum for medical schools in terms of knowledge, skills and attitudes.[2] You are expected to develop professional attitudes while studying.

Summary

- GMC guidance advises that you must not use your position as a doctor to establish emotional relationships with your patients.
- Medical students are encouraged to develop professional attitudes and follow guidance appropriate to registered doctors.

Reading

- British Medical Association. www.bma.org.uk – go to ethics, then to doctor–patient relationships.
- Council on Ethical and Judicial Affairs, American Medical Association. Sexual misconduct in the practice of medicine. *JAMA* 1991; 266: 2742–875.
- General Medical Council. *Good Medical Practice*. London: GMC, 2001.
- Hill J. Rules for romance. *Lancet* 2003; 361: 440.

References

1. General Medical Council. *Good Medical Practice*. London: GMC, May 2001. www.gmc_uk.org/standards/good.htm
2. General Medical Council. *Tomorrow's Doctors.* London: GMC, 2002.

CASE 19: PERFORMING INTIMATE EXAMINATIONS

Issues

Changing patient attitudes
Investigation of allegations and rumours
Bullying and harassment
Obtaining consent for examinations
Students in operating theatres as assistants
Patients who lack competence
Liability when no consent is obtained
Admission of errors to patients and apologies

Part 1

You are the clinical dean of your medical school. Last night at a social event, you heard on the medical grapevine that one of your consultant surgical colleagues in a nearby teaching hospital is bullying third-year students into carrying out intimate examinations of patients under general anaesthetic. The patients have not consented to these examinations.

One of your students comes to see you this morning, and bursts into tears as she tells you a similar story. She is deeply upset about it and feels guilty. She is talking about tracking down the patient to apologise personally for (in her words) 'assaulting her like that'.

- **What should you say to the student?**
- **How do you deal with the situation – do you:**
  - **investigate?**
  - **inform others in the faculty?**
  - **inform the GMC?**

Use this page to write down your own ideas

Changing patient attitudes

This case raises a topical issue in the area of medical education. Historically, medical students were often taught by methods which 'used' patients as 'subjects'. Patients were more 'learned on' than 'learned from'. Patients didn't always know what was happening, partly because 'what they didn't know wouldn't hurt them'.

Ways of thinking have changed. Patients now expect to be involved in their care, and as part of this they want to know how and when they can help the training of future doctors. Many patients are delighted to help. However, they want to be informed of what is happening to them.

Investigation of allegations and rumours

Hospitals and medical schools are close 'communities'. Rumours develop and circulate around such communities with amazing frequency. The question is, when do you ignore a rumour; when do you pass it on to your friends; and when do you think, 'This doesn't sound right, I'd better do something about this'? The answer to these questions will probably depend on the circumstances, and on the details of the rumour.

✿ What would you do if you heard a rumour about a friend or colleague?

A new Act of Parliament came into force in 1998 in the UK called the 'Public Interest Disclosure Act' (but commonly known as the 'Whistle-Blowing Act'). This was designed to protect employees by protecting anybody who 'blew the whistle' (informed the authorities) on a colleague from being victimised or dismissed.

Bullying and harassment

Bullying and harassment are defined as any persistent behaviour directed against an individual which is intimidating, offensive, or malicious, and which undermines the confidence and self-esteem of the recipient. The intimidating behaviour of a consultant threatening the students with expulsion from the firm certainly classifies as bullying under this or any other definition.

In a recent survey 37% of junior doctors report being bullied and 84% reported being bullied at some point in their career.[1] Bullying and harassment can take many forms: racial or sexual, explicit or implicit, verbal or physical, vertical or horizontal. The intimidation described in the above scenario falls clearly within the remit of unacceptable behaviour. Opinions differ on how to tackle inappropriate behaviour within the workplace and different people may have personal practices depending on their personalities and how they get on with the people concerned. Sometimes a quiet word expressing concern may be appropriate. If, however, as in this case, that is clearly insufficient, more formal procedures should be followed.

When reporting unacceptable behaviour, every trust should have guidelines in place. Occupational health should be available to support bullying and harassment claims. Every trust should also have whistle-blowing guidelines in place. The most important things to bear in mind are documentation and not being afraid to inform a senior person rather than informal colleagues. Your claim deserves to be taken seriously by others and by yourself. The BMA, as your trade union, should defend you in such cases (in July 2004 they were considering draft guidance on preventing such behaviour) and there may be implications with the GMC rules on fitness to practise for the other party.

In this case, it may be appropriate for the students to say something at the time of the offence, but if this is not possible due to the nature of the intimidation, then reporting should certainly take place after the event via the mechanisms described above.

Obtaining consent for examinations

Did you know that it is illegal to 'touch' a person without their consent? Doing so constitutes an act of assault. There are exceptions to this in medicine, such as when a patient is brought unconscious into an emergency department and they are unable to give consent, but as a general rule you *must* obtain consent before you examine anybody.

Consent does not necessarily need to be written down. A patient can imply that they give consent, eg offering you their arm when you ask to take blood from them. Consent can also be given verbally by a patient. In practice, doctors tend to formalise the procedure of obtaining consent by asking patients to sign a form. Although this is legally no better than a verbal agreement, it lends weight to the process, ensures that it has been done and provides evidence if necessary.

✿ What do you need to do to obtain valid consent from a patient for an examination or procedure?

✱ Consent must be given by a competent individual (see Case 2) and should be both voluntary and informed in order to be valid.

The Department of Health has issued guidelines about obtaining consent, which state that, ideally, the person who will perform the procedure should obtain consent from the patient.[2] Because this is not always possible in a busy hospital environment, doctors can delegate this task to somebody who is trained and understands the procedure, including its possible side-effects and complications.

Advice for obtaining informed consent

As a junior doctor, particularly in surgery, you will be required to obtain informed consent from patients. The GMC gives advice on this in *Seeking Patients' Consent*.[3] When doing this you should make the patient aware:

- of why the procedure is being proposed and the alternatives (including the option not to treat)
- of what will happen during the procedure
- of whether it will take place under sedation or local/general anaesthetic
- significant risks and complications (ie risks that are significant in the percentage of patients they affect (eg pain is a common problem), or in their nature (eg impotence, and death are serious consequences))
- proposed pre-procedure requirements (eg fasting) and post-procedure care (eg bed rest, catheters, drains)
- prognosis, including possible outcomes, findings and diagnoses
- that it may not be you who does the procedure
- that anything unnecessary will not be done
- that anything necessary will be done unless they specifically say that there is something they do not want to be done
- that they may ask any questions at any time
- that they may change their mind at any time
- of the extent to which students or doctors in training may be involved in the procedure.

Intimate examinations

What is an 'intimate' examination? You may believe that all examinations are intimate, as they involve an individual allowing their doctor (or a student) to touch them. Certain examinations require added respect however, as they involve a greater invasion of the patient's personal space. These examinations include those of the rectum, groin, breast, internal examinations in women and examinations of the male genitalia.

✿ What is different about performing an intimate examination, compared with any other examination?

To perform an intimate examination you need to go through the same procedure of obtaining consent as you would for any other examination of a person. The fact that you may find it a slightly embarrassing subject to talk about does not exclude you from asking the patient's permission.

✿ What can you think of that a patient may want to know before giving their consent for you to perform a procedure?

✿ Should a chaperone always be offered? For whom is the chaperone present? Can anyone act as a chaperone?

If you are a medical student in the case of an intimate examination, you may want to ensure that the following points have been emphasised – that:

- you are a medical student
- you are the student who will be doing the examination
- you will be doing it as an educational exercise
- you will be supervised by a qualified member of staff
- the examination will also be performed for diagnostic purposes by a doctor
- they do not have to give consent, and that, if they would prefer not to be involved, their own medical care will not be affected.

Examinations under anaesthetic

You may be given the opportunity to perform intimate examinations on patients while they are anaesthetised for an operation. Some people consider this to be a valuable experience as it allows students to become confident at recognising 'normal' as well as 'abnormal', while at the same time removing any possible embarrassment or unnecessary pain for the patient. Such examinations are not exempted from the need to obtain consent from the patient. In fact, the very nature of the examination, coupled with the patient's lack of awareness at the time of the event, makes it all the more important that you ask permission when the patient is awake, and preferably when they have not got far more important things to worry about!

Students in operating theatres as assistants

Assisting at an operation can be a very enjoyable and valuable learning experience for junior doctors and medical students.

✿ Usually, an assistant in theatre would examine the area of the body that is being operated upon. This may involve performing an intimate examination. If you are a student and you are asked to do this, what should you do about obtaining consent? Or is this just part of the job of the assistant?

This is a question asked by many, and it is a difficult one to answer. Strictly speaking, doctors should not depend on the examination findings of medical students. They should therefore repeat any examination that a student performs to confirm the findings. This essentially means that anything you do as a medical student is being done for your own educational purposes and not for the benefit of the patient. If this is the case, then you must obtain consent for any examination you perform on a patient.

Regarding assisting operations in general, it is good practice to meet the patient before you perform any surgery on them. Doctors (surgeons and anaesthetists) introduce themselves to their patients, so why shouldn't you as a student? If you spend some time chatting to them before their operation they will often ask if you will be watching. Even if they do not ask, you can always say to them, 'As long as it's okay with you, I'll be watching the op, and I'll pop back to say "Hi" when you come round afterwards.' A discussion such as this can easily be extended to discuss assisting the surgeon. A patient approached in this manner is usually delighted to help (and actually glad to know someone will be watching who can come and tell them all the juicy details about how it went afterwards!).

Patients who lack competence

✿ What do you remember about assessing a patient's competence? (See Cases 2 and 4.)

✿ How should you best treat a patient who is not competent to give consent to a procedure? Should incompetent patients ever be involved in education?

You may be able to think of situations where patients are not competent (for example, after an accident), but where you really need to treat them now if they are to have any chance of survival. It is possible for doctors to treat without consent in situations like this, as long as the treatment is deemed to be in the best interests of the patient (*F v West Berkshire HA* [1989] All ER 545).

✿ Under what circumstances (if any) do you think it is acceptable for a medical student to perform a physical examination on a patient who lacks competence to give consent? What about an intimate examination?

Liability when no consent is obtained

Matters such as these have not been tested in the courts in the UK, so the following points are purely speculative. If a person performs an act without first having obtained valid informed consent they risk facing criminal prosecution for assault and/or a civil action (trespass to the person or negligence). In addition, given the nature of intimate examinations, there is the possibility that someone could be charged with an offence under the Sexual Offences Act 2003. For a criminal charge, it is the individual who would be charged and possibly even convicted. For the civil wrongs, there might also be individual liability. However in the case of an NHS employee, the trust for which the individual worked could also be held 'vicariously' liable. (In the case of medical students, the university and medical school could be vicariously liable.)

Medical students are not solely responsible for their actions. If they are instructed to carry out a procedure by a doctor, the doctor has some responsibility for the outcomes that arise. This means that if you perform an examination without consent, the doctor who supervises you is also liable to charges of assault. As well as the issue of assault, there is a chance of supervising doctors being held negligent following cases of examinations on anaesthetised patients. A patient under anaesthetic is (albeit temporarily) incompetent to give consent.

♣ When a patient is not competent, the role of the doctor is to administer medical treatment that is considered necessary and in the best interests of the patient.

✿ Can you think of any situations where an educational examination by a student on a patient who has not given consent is in the best interests of that patient?

A doctor who does not act in the best interests of an incompetent patient may be found negligent.

Admission of errors to patients and apologies

The student concerned in this case considered informing the patient of what had happened.

✿ What would you do if you were placed in a similar position? Would you inform the patient? What would you tell them?

Defence organisations agree that if doctors showed empathy towards patients' complaints and apologised for mistakes, the amount of litigation against the medical profession would drop significantly. Apologising to a patient may make them feel better and may not necessarily be an admission of guilt on your part. Even simple apologies, such as, 'I'm sorry you have had to wait so long' or 'I'm sorry that you feel you have not been well looked after', can go a long way to helping patients feel that they have been listened to and therefore reduce the likelihood that they will put in a complaint.

The benefits of patients' complaints are only now being appreciated. The vast majority of complaints to complaint authorities and hospitals relate to *diagnosis and treatment*. These are not usually the 'fault' of any one person but a result of the *system* of care in which patients are treated. While a patient may complain about a particular medical student or doctor, an analysis of the complaint will usually discover many factors involved in the patient's care and treatment. Some doctors think a defensive attitude is the best approach to complaints, but studies show that patients are more likely to complain and sue doctors when there is no apology or open communication.

Why do patients complain?

- Because they are not given enough detail when consenting for a proposed treatment. It is best to provide patients with appropriate information and allow patients time to ask questions.
- Because some patients feel ignored by those responsible for their care and treatment after an adverse event takes place. If detailed explanations about what happened, why it happened and what will be done to help them overcome the problems were provided in a *timely* manner patients would not complain.
- Because some patients who receive substandard care are not provided with an *apology* for the inadequacies in the health service.
- Because some health providers do not afford patients dignity and treat them courteously.
- Because some doctors are poor communicators and fail to provide sufficient information and empathy to patients at a time of great vulnerability.

How do complaints help improve medicine?

- They lead to *improvements in practice*. Clinical decision-making and patient management comprise multiple tasks and complex processes. There is ample room for error. Complaints can identify particular parts of the process that require review.

- They help to *maintain standards*. They are one of the ways to identify doctors who are incompetent or unethical. A complaint by a patient can indicate that something may be wrong.
- They provide an *alternative to litigation*. Most complainants want an explanation about what happened, why it happened and assurances that it won't happen again. If a complaint is taken seriously by the hospital or doctor the complainant is unlikely to seek legal redress.
- They help maintain *public trust*. Complaints offer patients opportunities to have their concern about their care examined, but also it acts as a safety valve for other patients if the clinician is practising beyond their limits.
- They *encourage self-assessment*. Many complaints reflect inadequate communication. Complaints can cause doctors to re-evaluate their communication skills.
- They *remind doctors of their ethical and professional obligations*. The stress of receiving a complaint is well documented. Without complaints the vocational underpinnings of medicine would become weaker. If professionalism weakens so too does the medical profession.

What should you do if you receive a complaint?

You *will* make mistakes. You are human. Mistakes and complaints are prime learning opportunities and you should view them in this light. Hospitals are complex organisations involving many people in the care of patients, so if you receive a complaint the chances are that other factors will also be involved other than your care and treatment. Poor supervision, tiredness, and inexperience are all factors that contribute to mistakes but these are not the 'fault' of the individual at the point of care resulting in a complaint.

The following are golden rules, which will help you manage complaints and mistakes.

- You should discuss the complaint with your supervisor (clinical tutor, term supervisor, registrar)
- Never lie. If you made a mistake or you don't know what you did it is best to talk it over with your supervisor and he or she will help you understand the issues and help identify remedies. Be frank and honest about what you did and why.
- You should seek out information about how you could avoid repeating the error or conduct that led to the complaint.

- You should speak directly with the patient if appropriate. Apologise if appropriate and let the patient know what you have done to fix the problem.
- The medical records should be appropriately documented.

When a patient suffers a serious adverse event?

- Express sympathy and compassion to the patient or the family. (This will often diffuse a potentially volatile situation.)
- Do not take a defensive position and refrain from castigation or infighting with other members of the healthcare team.
- Do not accept or assign blame or criticise the care or response of other providers.
- Before you make a record in the medical notes discuss the circumstances with an appropriate supervisor.
- Keep the documentation to factual statements of the event and any follow-up required or done as a result of the incident.
- Avoid writing in the record any information unrelated to the care of the patient.
- As a junior doctor or medical student you will not be expected to manage the complaint or adverse events alone. Registrars or your supervisors will take the lead in discussions with the patients making the complaint or family members. You can use this opportunity to learn about communications with patients. Observe what works well and what does not.

Part 2

Two weeks later, another woman patient finds out that an illegal intimate examination has been performed on her during an exploratory operation, this time by two male medical students, under the direction of the same surgical consultant. One of the operating department practitioners (ODP) was a neighbour of the patient, and was shocked to see her examined without any apparent consent. The ODP told the woman what had happened, including the fact that the consultant had threatened the students with expulsion from his firm if they failed to examine the woman as demanded of them.

Think about this one yourself, and try to consider what action you may have taken if you had been the ODP.

- **Should it make any difference if the patient is your friend or relative?**
- **Would you have spoken up in the operating theatre in defence of the students?**
- **How might you go about raising concerns in a situation such as this?**

Summary

- Performing any examination without consent could result in criminal prosecution for assault or a civil action.
- Obtaining informed consent is an in-depth procedure, which involves giving information about what you are going to do and about any risks involved.
- Examinations carried out by students, and those done when patients are under anaesthetic must be done with consent, just like any other examination.
- Apologising to patients is not the same as admitting responsibility, and is recommended by defence organisations as an appropriate action following mistakes.

Reading

- Chartered Institute of Personnel Management quick fact and information sheets. *Bullying,* available at www.cipd.co.uk/infosource/HealthAndSafety/Bullying.asp; *Harassment,* available at www.cipd.co.uk/infosource/EqualityandDiversity/Harassment.asp
- Coldicott Y, Pope C, Roberts C. The ethics of intimate examinations – teaching tomorrow's doctors. *BMJ* 2003; 326: 97–101.
- Coull R. Everything you always wanted to know about whistle-blowing but were afraid to ask. *BMJ Career Focus* 2004; 328: s5–6.
- Cusack S. Workplace bullying: icebergs in sight, soundings needed. *Lancet* 2000; 356: 9248.
- Hickson GB, Clayton EW, Githens PB, Sloan FA. Factors that prompted families to file malpractice claims following perinatal injuries. *JAMA* 1992; 267: 1359–63.
- Hingorani M, Wong T, Vafidis G. Patients' and doctors' attitudes to amount of information given after unintended injury during treatment: cross-sectional, questionnaire survey. *BMJ* 1999; 318: 640–1.
- Huycke L, Huycke M. Characteristics of potential plaintiffs on malpractice. *Annals of Internal Medicine* 1994; 120(9): 792–8.
- Flynn S, Rossiter A. Bullying and harassment at work. *BMJ Career Focus* 2003; 327: s164–5.

- Penchansky R, Macnee C. Initiation of medical malpractice suits: a conceptualization and test. *Med Care* 1994; 32: 813–31
- Quine L. Workplace bullying in junior doctors: questionnaire survey. *BMJ* 2002; 324: 878–9.
- Special issue of *BMJ Career Focus* devoted to tackling bullying. http://bmj.com/content/vol326/issue7393/#CAREER
- Vincent C, Young M, Phillips A. Why do people sue doctors? A study of patients and relatives taking legal action. *Lancet* 1994; 343(8913): 1609–13.
- Witman AB, Park DM, Hardin SB. How do patients want physicians to handle mistakes? A survey of internal medicine patients in an academic setting. *Archives of Internal Medicine* 1996; 156(22): 2565–9.

References

1. Quine L. Workplace bullying in junior doctors: questionnaire survey. *BMJ* 2002; 324: 878–9.
2. Department of Health. *Reference Guide to Consent for Examination or Treatment.* London: Department of Health, 2001.
3. General Medical Council. *Seeking Patients' Consent.* London: GMC, 1998.

CASE 20: PROFESSIONAL COURTESY AND FOUL PLAY

Issues

Cheating and plagiarism
Reporting concerns about colleagues
Queue jumping

You are an SpR in orthopaedics. Your best friend from medical school is now starting his MD, also in orthopaedics. He visits you socially, and after a couple of drinks mentions that he is extremely upset as his research is going abysmally and he is getting no results whatsoever. He asks if he can see your work that you completed the previous year 'for inspiration'. You agree, and find out a couple of months later that the MD he's submitted is remarkably similar to yours.

- **What do you do?**
- **Who do you approach?**
- **What do you think about cheats?**
- **Do you think it is incompatible for doctors to be cheats, or can they cheat in exams and still be good doctors?**

A couple of years later, when you are a newly registered consultant, the same friend visits you following a rugby injury and asks you if you can squeeze him in for a knee arthroscopy. Your lists are already overbooked and any additional cases would delay someone else's treatment.

- **What would you say to him?**
- **Should NHS employees receive preferential treatment?**
- **Are there ethical justifications for NHS employees to be treated more quickly on the NHS?**

Use this page to write down your own ideas

Cheating and plagiarism

Research has shown that many medical students do cheat, in one form or another.[1] People have different ideas about what constitutes cheating.

✿ Think about the following. Do you think that they are forms of cheating?

- Forging your absent friend's signature on an attendance register, or forging your consultant's signature in a personal log of procedures you have performed.
- Copying your SSM from that of a friend at a different medical school.
- Copying an elective report from the Internet.
- Writing in the notes 'chest clear, respiratory rate 16, trachea central', but not actually performing an examination at all.

✿ Have you ever cheated? How did you feel about doing it? What were the consequences? What do you think would have happened if you had been found out?

✿ What is plagiarism? Is there a difference between plagiarism and cheating?

People can fool themselves into thinking that plagiarism is not cheating. However, plagiarism is a form of cheating and is always regarded as a serious offence. It can be avoided by ensuring that you reference all your work according to the guidelines laid out by your medical school/journal.

Reporting concerns about colleagues

✿ Your friend may be well known among his peers as someone who is of dubious character. Would you want to be associated with him if he was behaving unprofessionally? If you did associate with him, what do you think your other colleagues would think of you?

✿ How would you go about reporting your concerns?

The Public Interest Disclosure Act (Whistle-Blowing Act; see Cases 6 and 19) was established to make informing on poor conduct of work colleagues much easier.

Queue jumping

✿ Should doctors (and their families) receive preferential treatment on the NHS? For example, do you think they should jump the waiting list? Or should they always see a consultant in a clinic, and not a junior doctor?

It is generally thought that the queue jumping of doctors is 'unjust' in ethical terms and many trusts indicate in their code of conduct that employees must not seek preferential treatment on the NHS. The jumping of queues by employees is seen to occur at the expense of other patients.

South Devon Healthcare Trust caused controversy some years ago when it implemented a policy explicitly advocating the *opposite*, justifying it on ethical grounds. The trust's medical director justified it for three reasons: 'Firstly, we value our employees and want to do the best for them. Secondly, we want the trust to run as efficiently as possible to serve the public, and that means getting employees back to work quicker. Thirdly, this policy ensures that we save money on locums and other staff, who can cost hundreds of pounds a session.' Although this argument may apply to treatment that affects a doctor's ability to function, it is not really valid in an elective case such as an arthroscopy. Whatever the justification for a non-preferential (or a preferential) treatment policy by the trust, all employees should adhere to it.

Summary

Professional misconduct can occur more easily than you might think. Ignorance is not an excuse – always be prepared to justify your actions.

Reading

- Boulton A. Trust criticised for putting staff before patients. *BMJ* 1996; 312: 396–7.
- Rennie SC, Crosby JR. Are 'tomorrow's doctors' honest? Questionnaire study exploring medical students' attitudes and reported behaviour on academic misconduct. *BMJ* 2001; 322: 274–5.

Reference

1. Rennie SC, Crosby JR. Are 'tomorrow's doctors' honest? Questionnaire study exploring medical students' attitudes and reported behaviour on academic misconduct. *BMJ* 2001; 322: 274–5.

CASE 21: IS THERE SUCH A THING AS A FREE LUNCH?

Issues

Professional obligations
Autonomous decisions – the choice of individuals

You are a senior house officer on a medical firm. The mess president has organised a drug representative to host a meal for all the junior doctors. One of your friends says that she has a conscientious objection to going as in her opinion the meal is just a form of bribery for which patients will bear the cost. However, you do not agree as you do not have any influence over prescribing policy (hospital pharmacy and your consultant determine that) and, besides, it will be a very sociable occasion, so you put your name down.

- What contacts have you had so far with the pharmaceutical industry?
- Have you ever felt compromised ethically by these contacts?
- Are you aware of any guidance for doctors as to what is and what is not appropriate?
- How would you decide what kind of drug-sponsored function was appropriate to attend?

Use this page to write down your own ideas

Professional obligations

'Can't live with 'em, can't live without 'em.' The relationship between the pharmaceutical industry and the medical profession has long been one of mutual dependence characterised by a delicate balance between flattery and distrust. As commercial corporations, pharmaceutical companies have the primary aim, indeed legal obligation, to increase profit for their shareholders. Most would agree that the best way of selling pharmaceuticals and increasing revenue is by producing high-quality products that are effective in trials and benefit the patient. To evaluate which of the pharmaceutical products available on the market are best suited to the needs of their patients, doctors consult a variety of sources: journals and reviews, hospital protocols, advice from seniors and colleagues, and, whether acknowledged or not, promotions by pharmaceutical companies. These companies represent a multi-million-pound industry and this presents the following ethical problems:

- **Beneficence** – The doctor's role is to act as the patient's advocate, and this also applies in dealing with pharmaceutical companies. While many may make claims to the contrary, it has been shown that doctors' prescribing practice *is* influenced by gifts from pharmaceutical companies[1] and this clearly compromises a doctor's capacity to act entirely in the best interests of the patient.
- **Non-maleficence** – Gifts from pharmaceutical companies are taken out of the company's profits which have to be recovered in the cost of the drug, which will be borne by the NHS and the patient through decreased NHS funding as a result.
- **Distributive justice** – The costs borne by the NHS due to the increased costs of a particular type of drug may adversely affect the resources allocated to a particular group of patients.
- **Doctor–patient relationship** – In accepting gifts from pharmaceutical companies, the doctors ceases to be an unbiased representative of the patient. At best, he or she becomes a broker, at worst a thief.

Guidance

Although limited guidance had existed for some time, namely by the Association of British Pharmaceutical Industries, persistent transgressions prompted the government to ban expensive gifts such as holidays, cash and equipment for personal use in parliamentary regulation in 1994.[2] In 2002, the Royal College of Physicians, London updated its 1986 guidelines on the same subject and greatly refined the conditions under which gifts may be accepted by doctors. These stated that gifts, hospitality and 'kind' should be directly or indirectly educational, they should be declared, no conditions must be attached to them and they should not be extended to spouses.[3] This reflects an international tightening of the regulation of pharmaceutical gifts and warns of the possible prosecution of doctors and companies that have violated them.[4]

The American Medical Student Association advocates an amendment to the Hippocratic Oath to include a commitment to 'make medical decisions . . . free from the influence of advertising or promotion. I will not accept money, gifts, or hospitality that will create a conflict of interest in my education, practice, teaching, or research.'[5]

Autonomous decisions – the choice of individuals

So much for guidance, but how do individual doctors and medical students decide their ethical stance in a particular situation? The No Free Lunch organisation light-heartedly advocates each doctor or medical student to take an adapted 'drug rep dependence' CAGE questionnaire after the alcohol dependence questionnaire of the same name.

- Have you ever prescribed **C**elebrex?
- Been **A**nnoyed by people who complain about drug lunches?
- Is there a medication lo**G**o on the pen you're using?
- Do you drink your morning **E**ye-opener out of a Fastab mug?

This may be somewhat facetious but the idea may be close to the truth in that within the given guidelines and based on the principles, *both* you and your friend may be right in your respective decisions of attending or not attending the meal.

Summary
- The pharmaceutical and medical professions are inevitably interlinked, but often have different agendas.
- All four major ethical principles are at stake when the medical and pharmaceutical professions interact.
- Professional guidance says you should limit gifts to an absolute minimum.

Reading
- Bennett J, Collins J. The relationship between physicians and the biomedical industries: advice from the Royal College of Physicians. *Clinical Medicine* 2002; 2: 320–2.

- General Medical Council. The duties of a doctor registered with the general medical council. www.gmc-uk.org
- McGuaran A. Royal College issues new guidelines on gifts from drug companies. *BMJ* 2002; 325: 511.
- Moynihan R. Who pays for the pizza? Redefining the relationships between doctors and drug companies. 2: Disentanglement. *BMJ* 2003; 326: 1193–6.
- Wazana A. Physicians and the pharmaceutical industry: is a gift ever just a gift? *JAMA* 2000; 283: 373–80.

References

1. Wazana A. Physicians and the pharmaceutical industry: is a gift ever just a gift? *JAMA* 2000; 283: 373–80.
2. Beecham L. Government acts on gifts from drug companies. *BMJ* 1994; 309: 292.
3. Bennett J, Collins J. The relationship between physicians and the biomedical industries: advice from the Royal College of Physicians. *Clinical Medicine* 2002; 2: 320–2. [Q26]
4. McGuaran A. Royal College issues new guidelines on gifts from drug companies. *BMJ* 2002; 325: 511.
5. Moynihan R. Who pays for the pizza? Redefining the relationships between doctors and drug companies. 2: Disentanglement. *BMJ* 2003; 326: 1193–6.

CASE 22: PUBLICATION ETHICS, DATA PROTECTION AND FREEDOM OF INFORMATION

Issues

Publication ethics

You are in a relationship with a drug representative called Sally. By complete coincidence, you find out that one of the drugs you are researching is produced by another subsidiary of Sally's drug company. Sally has some shares in this company but as you are not married you do not think you have any obligation to declare this link – besides, you did not even know of it at the time of doing the research and you fear that declaring this will unfairly discredit your research.

■ **What are the relationships between pharmaceutical companies and medical research and what are the ethical issues involved?**
■ **Can you think of any potential and real conflicts of interest and to what extent are they important for others to know about?**
■ **Is sponsored science bad science?**

As part of your research you have accessed 1352 patient records. Sally asks you if she could look into some of the patient records to see what drugs have been prescribed for them. She says it would not cause any harm and there would be no consequences (except for making her life a lot easier). She says she should be able to see them under the new Freedom of Information Act which makes NHS documents public.

■ **Is she right in thinking there would be no adverse consequences to such actions?**
■ **Is she correct in her interpretation of the Freedom of Information Act?**
■ **What are the ethical and legal principles behind data protection for (i) research and (ii) commercial purposes?**

Use this page to write down your own ideas

Publication ethics

Pharmaceutical industry interests are as entwined with the medical researchers as they are with clinicians. Examples include paid speaking arrangements, consultancies and positions on advisory boards, as well as equity earnings – all of which are potentially extremely lucrative.[1]

The Committee on Publication Ethics (COPE) was formed in 1997 by the editors of leading medical journals and issues guidance on all aspects of publication ethics, including conflicts of interest. Their guidelines state clearly that 'when in doubt, disclose'.[2] Dr Andrew Wakefield's trial on MMR was discredited by the *Lancet* editor, Richard Horton when it was discovered that Wakefield was being paid to carry out a similar trial to support the compensation claims of children with autism.[3] Although the conflict of interests in this case may not have affected the research, being seen to be fair is as important as actually being fair, and transparency is to be recommended.

A patient's medical notes comprise a very private record, containing many details pertaining to many areas of their life and oftentimes their family. Although common law is not developed in a very logical way, these records are protected in both statutory and quasi-legal frameworks.

General Medical Council guidance

The GMC[4] advises that doctors should minimise disclosure of confidential information, and that when they do the information should be made anonymous. The patient should be informed and express written consent should be obtained wherever feasible; certainly for use of confidential information outside research and audit, especially when the patient is identifiable. Information shared within teams is permissible but should be respected. See below the relevant paragraphs:[4]

- 'Where patients have consented to treatment, express consent is not usually needed before relevant personal information is shared to enable treatment to be provided.' (paragraph 7)
- 'You should make sure that patients are aware that personal information about them will be shared within the healthcare team unless they object, and the reasons for this.' (paragraph 8)
- 'Anyone to whom personal information is disclosed in confidence must respect that confidence.' (paragraph 9)
- 'Disclosure for use in education or training, clinical or medical audit is unlikely to have personal consequences for the patient. In these circumstances you should still obtain patients' express consent to the

use of identifiable data or arrange for members of the healthcare team to anonymise records.' (paragraph 15)

Data Protection Act 1998

This Act provides the basis of the statute on data protection. It applies to both computer and manual records. It defines eight principles which broadly state that data should be processed fairly, securely, and for limited purposes. It is under this Act that patients have a right to view their records, subject to a prescribed fee, although data holders are not obliged to release information pertaining to a third party or information that may harm the patient.

Access to medical records for research purposes should in theory also be covered by the Data Protection Act, although there is a lot of uncertainty about the nature of how it is covered. The GMC initially warned that putting a patient on the cancer registry might constitute a breach of the Act – now it seems that with appropriate anonymity, the use of personal records for research and audit is permissible.

Freedom of Information Act 2000

This Act, implemented in January 2005, gives a right of access to information held by public bodies, including the NHS. It does not, however, cover access to personal information, eg medical records, and certainly not that of other people. It gives access about details of the running of the NHS, including policies such as resource allocation. Many NHS trusts have issued 'publication schemes' to address the responsibilities imposed by the Freedom of Information Act.

It is not yet fully known to what extent the media will use this Act to acquire information to be used in big media 'scares', such as methicillin-resistant *Staphylococcus aureus* (MRSA) or meningitis outbreaks. Public bodies are not obliged to give out all information, and it is likely that NHS bodies will still be able to protect themselves against the manipulation of facts by the media.

Other aspects of confidentiality are discussed in Case 1 including the permissible exceptions. These do not apply to the supply of medical notes to pharmaceutical companies for marketing purposes and therefore you are legally and morally obliged to protect confidentiality as prescribed by the Data Protection Act 1998 – regardless of your personal relationships.

Summary

- Always declare any real or potential conflicts of interest when publishing. Your career may not survive to regret it if you do not.
- Patients' medical notes are protected by statute in the form of the Data Protection Act and the Human Rights Act, and by GMC guidance.
- Patients have access to medical information by means of the Data Protection Act and the Freedom of Information Act.

Reading

- Committee on Publication Ethics (COPE). Guidelines on good publication practice. www.publicationethics.org
- General Medical Council. Confidentiality: Protecting and Providing Information and Research: The Roles and Responsibilities of Doctors. www.gmc-uk.org
- General Medical Council. Duties of the Doctor and Ethical Research: The Roles and Responsibilities of Doctors. www.gmc-uk.org
- Horton R. The lessons of MMR. *Lancet* 2004; 363: 1473–4.
- Meredith B. Data protection and the freedom of information. *BMJ* 2005; 330: 490–1.
- Moynihan R. Who pays for the pizza? Redefining the relationships between doctors and drug companies. 2: Disentanglement *BMJ* 2003; 326: 1193–6.
- Peto J, Fletcher O, Gilham C. Data protection, informed consent, and research. *BMJ* 2004; 328: 1029–30.

References

1. Moynihan R. Who pays for the pizza? Redefining the relationships between doctors and drug companies. 2: Disentanglement *BMJ* 2003; 326: 1193–6.
2. Committee on Publication Ethics (COPE). Guidelines on good publication practice. www.publicationethics.org
3. Horton R. The lessons of MMR. *Lancet* 2004; 363: 1473–4.
4. General Medical Council. *Confidentiality: Protecting and Providing Information.* London: GMC, 2004.

CASE 23: MEDICINE IN THE DEVELOPING WORLD – ELECTIVE ETHICS?

Issues

Professional obligations for medical students
Universality of ethical principles – global research, global ethics
Doctors and torture
Consequentialism versus deontology

You are a final-year medical student with an interest in tropical medicine, so you choose to do your elective in Uganda. While there you find yourself in a tiny rural hospital with virtually no facilities and an enormous number of patients. On one shift there is only one Ugandan doctor, who has asked you to help with several urgent lumbar punctures on a number of patients suspected of being victims of a meningitis outbreak. You have learnt how to perform lumbar punctures in clinical skills training and have observed many being done but have never actually done one yourself.

- **What do you do?**

After several weeks in the hospital you prove yourself to be a useful and competent member of the hospital team and you gain a lot of respect. A patient comes in with suspected appendicitis. The surgical registrar says that you should take the opportunity of being in Uganda to gain as much experience as possible and encourages you to do the operation. You know that in the UK only qualified doctors with several years' experience start to undertake operations.

- **What are the ethical duties of medical students on electives?**
- **How do you determine your boundaries?**
- **What steps might you take to complete your elective without seriously compromising your ethical standards?**
- **Can you justify doing an appendicectomy, under-qualified, for the sake of helping other patients better in the future?**

As part of your elective project you are required to participate in some research. You are invited to join the research of one of the local doctors who, in collaboration with an American pharmaceutical company, is looking to test a radical new antiretroviral therapy. The researchers have randomised a group of HIV-negative commercial sex workers into two groups and have developed a pessary cream. They would like to give the cream to one of the two groups and a placebo to the other. They plan to calculate if, after three months, the number of women using the pessary cream who have contracted HIV is statistically significantly less than in the placebo group. When you challenge the doctor about the ethics of this research, he says that 'women like that' would not use condoms anyway and that, this way, at least half the women will have some protection which they would not otherwise have, as well as enjoying the satisfaction of helping to devise a potentially valuable new preventive method for HIV infection. You notice that the consent sheets are all in English, which the local women are unable to read.

- **What are the potential benefits and harms of doing research in the developing world for**
  - **the subjects?**
  - **researchers? and**
  - **other parties?**
- **Are ethical principles universal and how does this relate to medical research?**
- **What factors influence the quality of informed consent with regard to research taking place in the developing world?**
- **How should research be regulated and monitored?**

Another patient in the hospital is brought in by the police with lots of fresh wounds. You ascertain that the police are holding him on 'terrorism charges', claiming that he is a rebel from nearby Rwanda. You suspect that he is being tortured by the police.

- **What do you do?**
- **Do you think torture can ever be justified?**
- **Do you feel medical practitioners have any special obligations towards prisoners, compared with the general population?**
- **Would you act differently as a student, than as you would if you were a qualified professional?**

Use this page to write down your own ideas

Professional obligations for medical students

First, do no harm

The key themes in these examples is whether, within your capabilities, the best interests of your patient are your first concern as required by the Hippocratic Oath, the GMC 'duties of the doctor' guidance and the World Medical Association Declaration of Geneva. Many of these ethical guides have originated in the developed world, and this has oftentimes led to accusations of imperialism in knowledge. It could be argued that this should indicate a need to involve the developed world more actively in the development of ethical guidance, rather than serve as an excuse to apply these principles selectively in a way which is often exploitative of people in the developed world.

Physician, know thy limits

In the first clinical example, you have never done a lumbar puncture but you are capable of doing one with your available knowledge and skills. To do one would be doing more good than harm, although you should request supervision until you feel confident to do the procedure independently.

In the second clinical example, you have never done the procedure before either, but the situation is radically different. Here you are not capable of doing it – you do not possess the necessary knowledge of anatomy and the skills of surgery. To do the procedure here would be doing more harm than good. The argument that you by doing the appendicectomy would gain knowledge and thereby benefit future patients is not valid – there are other, more effective ways to learn surgical skills which are appropriate to your level of training, such as learning to suture or assisting in the operation in other ways.

While it is important to take advantage of *appropriate* clinical experience, whether in the UK or overseas, you should always seek supervision and training when not entirely confident about a procedure.

Universality of ethical principles – global research, global ethics

As globalisation continues into the twenty-first century, so do issues relating to research ethics. Many researchers see the developing world as an opportunity to develop trials of new drugs. Although there is nothing inherently wrong with this premise, it does leave the door wide open for ethical problems. Potential benefits of research taking place in developing countries include:

■ **For the subjects** – For many people in the developing world, therapeutic trials offer the only chance of gaining access to drugs. In addition, financial inducements and other incentives for individuals and communities, far from being seen as exploitative are seen as hugely beneficial.

■ **For the researchers in the developing world** – Collaboration with researchers from the developed world is hugely beneficial in terms of building of local capacity and the sharing and procurement of equipment and knowledge, including ethical knowledge.

■ **For the researchers from the developed world** – Trials taking place in the developing world have been deemed to be hugely beneficial for the science community, largely because of the ability to generate huge numbers in trials, and the lack of bureaucratic hurdles. As the ethical issues around research ethics are being addressed, the relative benefits decline, yet the developing world is still seen as a fertile research area.

Potential harmful effects of research taking place in developing countries include:

■ **Standards of care** – It is stipulated that in clinical trials drugs should be tried against the 'best proven alternative diagnostic and therapeutic method'.[1] This has often served as an excuse to trial drugs against a placebo, as there is often no freely available alternative treatment to many diseases in the developing world. The universality of ethical principles and ethical standards (Council for International Organizations of Medical Sciences (CIOMS), *International Ethical Guidelines for Biomedical Research Involving Human Subjects*) would dictate that the next best alternative treatment should be that available in the marketplace, whether or not it is actually accessible to the subjects. This protects subjects in the developing world from exploitation by Western researchers. These principles were consolidated following the controversy surrounding the vertical transmission HIV trials in South Africa in the early 1990s.[2]

■ **Quality of consent** – Consent is often grossly inadequate in trials taking place in the developing world. Poor information due to issues around education further jeopardise the quality of consent.

What happens next?

If the trial is successful, will the procedure or drug be made available (i) to the original research subjects who might have experienced some benefit and/or (ii) in the community in which it was tested?

In the research proposal outlined above there is a great potential for harm. There is no prior evidence that this drug is safe for use in humans; and the standard against which the cream is tested is non-existent and the consent is of poor quality. The benefits of the research as outlined above are far outweighed by the potential harm to the subjects.

Research ethics committees are designed to protect the interests of the subject as well as facilitating research to benefit the community. There should be lay representation and continual review of protocols. It is important that all research involving human subjects, including research done by medical students, is approved by a research ethics committee, both in the country of the researcher and in the country in which the research is taking place.

Doctors and torture – ends and means

It is a cruel irony that because of their specialist skills which enable them to promote the health of humans, doctors are very frequently implicated in those acts which so utterly violate them. It was the crimes of Nazi doctors that inspired the first code of ethics in Nuremberg in 1947. Since then the World Medical Association issued a policy in Japan in 1975. Transgressions of the code signed up to by individual national medical associations are notable and often endemic within a group of the profession. So the Israeli Medical Association, for example, has come under heavy international condemnation for its participation in state policy to allow torture.[3] Similarly, more recently, the American medical profession has been implicated in human rights violations in Guantanamo Bay, Afghanistan and Iraq.[4]

The ethical justification for torture is often consequentialist in nature – namely that the end justifies the means. Whether or not this is a valid argument is outside the scope of this book although reference is made within the context of the Doctrine of Double Effect in Case 2. What is more important, however, is that it is a political and not a medical argument. As far as the medical profession is concerned, ethically and quasi-legally, doctors should not be complicit with any form of torture or abuse, and should endeavour to prevent it when at all possible. In the case above, the Tokyo Declaration would suggest that as a member of the medical profession the student should attempt to prevent the abuses against the prisoner – either by their documentation or their reporting. Nevertheless it is questionable whether there is an absolute duty to do so, especially if there were personal security implications.

Consequentialism versus deontology – now *you* decide

In order to protect your own code of ethical conduct on this otherwise valuable elective, you will need to clarify your boundaries with your Ugandan senior colleagues surrounding all these matters. Your seniors must be made aware that while you are there to learn, patients' lives and wellbeing must not be compromised.

Summary

- When in the developing world, you have to be more, rather than less aware of ethical principles.
- Research in the developing world has great potential benefits, but there is also much scope for exploitation.
- The medical profession should always protect the vulnerable in times of conflict, and distance itself from political pressures such as the 'war on terror', which may threaten Hippocratic principles.

Reading

- Central Office for Research Ethics Committees. Guidance for the REC community. www.corec.org.uk/recs/guidance/guidance
- Council for International Organizations of Medical Sciences (CIOMS). International ethical guidelines for biomedical research involving human subjects. www.cioms.ch/frame_guidelines_nov_2002
- General Medical Council. Duties of a doctor registered with the General Medical Council. www.gmc-uk.org
- Lurie P, Wolfe SM. Unethical trials of interventions to reduce perinatal transmission of the human immunodeficiency virus in developing countries. *New England Journal of Medicine* 1997; 337: 853–6.
- Miles SH. Abu Ghraib: its legacy for military medicine. *Lancet* 2004; 364: 724–9.
- Summerfield D. Israeli Medical Association shirks 'political aspects' of torture. *BMJ* 1995; 311: 755.

- World Medical Association. *Declaration of Geneva. Duties of a Medical Physician.* London: WMA, 1949. Adopted by the 3rd General Assembly of the World Medical Association, London, England, October 1949 and amended by the 22nd World Medical Assembly, Syndney, Australia, August 1968 and the 35th World Medical Assembly, Venice, Italy, October 1983.
- World Medical Association. *Declaration of Tokyo, Guidelines for Medical Doctors Concerning Torture and Other Cruel, Inhuman or Degrading Treatment or Punishment in Relation to Detention and Imprisonment.* Tokyo: WMA, 1975.
- World Medical Association. *Declaration of Helsinki, Ethical Principles for Medical Research Involving Human Subjects.* Adopted by the 18th WMA General Assembly, Helsinki, Finland, June 1964, and amended by the 52nd WMA General Assembly, Edinburgh, Scotland, October 2000.

References

1. World Medical Association. *Declaration of Helsinki, Ethical Principles for Medical Research Involving Human Subjects.* Adopted by the 18th WMA General Assembly, Helsinki, Finland, June 1964, and amended by the 52nd WMA General Assembly, Edinburgh, Scotland, October 2000.
2. Lurie P, Wolfe SM. Unethical trials of interventions to reduce perinatal transmission of the human immunodeficiency virus in developing countries. *New England Journal of Medicine* 1997; 337: 853–6.
3. Summerfield D. Israeli Medical Association shirks 'political aspects' of torture. *BMJ* 1995; 311: 755.
4. Miles SH. Abu Ghraib: its legacy for military medicine. *Lancet* 2004; 364: 724–9.

CASE 24: MEDICAL PRACTICE IN THE POST-SHIPMAN ERA

Issues

Keeping tabs? (Professional regulation)
Gifts from patients

You are an experienced GP in a rural practice. You have known Grace (aged 93) since you first joined the practice 23 years ago. You saw her in your surgery ten days previously and she was well, but she calls you and reports that she has a severe, dull pain radiating to her left arm. You call the ambulance and rush over to her house yourself but when you arrive she is dead. You are saddened but relieved that she died suddenly and having been in such good health previously. You cite 'myocardial infarction' as the cause of death on the certificate.

Grace's family are utterly dismayed at the news of her death. Her eldest son in particular is completely incredulous and accuses you of 'bumping her off' for financial gain. He cites as the fact that Grace always gave you a bottle of wine at Christmas as evidence. He reports that two more of your patients had died in the same month and says Grace's cause of death was never confirmed. 'Prove you're not like that Shipman fellow', he says.

- Should you have been completely sure of a cause of death before signing it on a death certificate?
- In what instances should you report a death to the coroner?
- What is the legacy of the Shipman Inquiry on medical practice?
- Do you think there is any benefit to be gained from monitoring GPs' mortality figures?
- Do you think current measures are adequate in protecting against future Shipmans?
- Is self-regulation appropriate in the medical profession?
- Do you think doctors should accept gifts from patients?

Use this page to write down your own ideas

Keeping tabs? (Professional regulation)

In the first report, the Shipman Inquiry (led by Dame Janet Smith) commissioned an independent team from Imperial College, London to look into mortality rates among patients registered with GPs. GPs with high mortality rates, however, were generally accounted for due to the 'nursing home effect' and were exonerated. This method is generally considered to be an unreliable 'screening' tool for picking out Shipmans and, although it could be used to back up other evidence, it should be discouraged as routine practice.

Reporting

In the third report, the Inquiry tackled the problem of death certification and reporting, especially in relation to cremation. This was tackled in more detail in Case 8. In the case outlined above, although the death was unexpected, it is doubtful whether it is suspicious to the extent of qualifying for referral by the above criteria. If you are in doubt then consult coroner's office for advice.

Regulation

On a background of changing perceptions and expectations of doctors, the Harold Shipman case catalysed a demand for greater openness in medical regulation. The GMC's statutory purpose is 'to protect, promote and maintain the health and safety of the public'. Following the scandals of the late 1990s, the GMC sought to introduce a revalidation scheme, with the primary purpose of making GMC registration more meaningful, and a subsidiary purpose of picking up 'problem doctors'.

The fifth report of the Shipman Inquiry strongly criticised the GMC for its failure to protect patients against Harold Shipman, pointing out his previous record of dishonest behaviour. The GMC has responded by streamlining its 'Fitness to Practise' procedures and have included more lay (non-medical) representation. It has also postponed its launch of the licensing and revalidation programme pending a government review of the Inquiry.

Gifts from patients

Doctors should be able to defend themselves against charges of financial exploitation of their patients. It is unethical for doctors to encourage patients to give them gifts. If a patient offers a gift of their own volition, then the nature of the gift should be considered. Something like a garment of underwear may be inappropriate, because of the sexual boundary it violates in the doctor–patient relationship. A substantial sum of money may be inappropriate because of the conflict of interests it may cause, which also compromises the doctor–patient relationship. Patients should instead donate substantial sums of money to a trust or charities rather than to individual doctors. Gifts such as a bottle of wine could arguably enhance the doctor–patient relationship by allowing the patient to express their gratitude and should not be regarded as inappropriate.

In March 2004 the BMA brought into force regulations specifying that a register should be kept of gifts from patients and their relatives which have a value of £100 or more (unless the gift is unrelated to the provision of service). The primary care trusts have access to this register.

If a patient wishes to bestow a substantial gift and the doctor deems the patient to lack capacity or be incompetent to give their consent freely, then it is advisable to have an independent third party present. A solicitor can verify that the doctor acted honourably when signing any documents on the patients' behalf.

Summary

As horrifically isolated an individual as Harold Shipman was, his crimes have left a scar on the public perception of the medical profession and have exposed weaknesses in the regulatory process, both of which must be addressed.

Reading

- The Shipman Inquiry. www.the-shipman-inquiry.org.uk/report
- Smith G. Dealing with deaths. *BMJ Career Focus* 2002; 325: 107.

CASE 25: MEDICINE IN THE AGE OF THE HUMAN RIGHTS ACT

Issues

Human Rights Act 1998

You are a urology consultant. One day you get a formal letter from one of your patients saying that he is taking you to court for assault and emotional trauma caused by a circumcision you performed on him 19 years ago. He claims you had violated article 3 of the Human Rights Act.

At the same time, you are enraged about the new consultant contract. You liaise with colleagues and attempt to make a claim under article 4 of the Human Rights Act.

- **What is the Human Rights Act?**
- **Do either of you have claims?**
- **What implications does the Act have for doctors?**

Use this page to write down your own ideas

Human Rights Act 1998

The Human Rights Act 1998 came into force in October 2000 in England and in other areas of the UK before this. It incorporates most of the European Convention of Human Rights which was set up after the Second World War and signed up to by 45 countries. Breaches of the Convention were previously brought to the ECHR in Strasbourg.

The Human Rights Act 1998 has two main practical implications: first, it brings the articles of the European Convention of Human Rights into UK law so that these cases can be tried in UK courts, and, second, it holds public authorities in this country accountable to its principles. The courts are encouraged to apply the law in a way which is consistent with the Act. Proceedings can be made by a person (including a private body, but not a public authority) against a public authority. The person, or 'victim', must be personally and directly affected by the breech; relatives can bring claims if the victim lacks capacity or is dead.

The aim of the Human Rights Act is to protect the rights of individuals from the potential tyranny of the majority. Critics of the Act will argue that protecting the rights of the individual will come at a cost to society. Apart from the principled, rights-based objections to the Act, there are also practical uncertainties in its interpretation. Definitions are usually quite vague, and what happens when there is a conflict between two different articles? Most of the articles are qualified; only articles 3 and 4 are absolute. In an editorial in the *Lancet*, Richard Horton explained the Human Rights Act's effects on the medical profession[1] (see following sections).

Article 2: Right to life

The first question to arise is: 'What is life'? Is an unborn child alive, and does abortion therefore violate this right? Is embryonic stem cell research a violation of article 2?

In relation to end-of-life decisions, the terminology is clearer, but the implications are not. Does a right to life automatically confer a right to death? Mrs Diane Pretty failed to claim this right at the European Court of Human Rights in Strasbourg (see Case 2). The Human Rights Act also does not offer assistance in cases when one person's life is dependent on another's as in the case of conjoined twins.

Article 3: Prohibition of torture and inhuman and degrading treatment

The very first cases heard under the new Human Rights Act in October 2000 were right-to-die cases on behalf of two patients in a persistent vegetative state. They were supported by this article and won. Mrs Diane Pretty brought a claim under this article of the Act in 2002 when she went to the House of Lords and failed. The man who contacted the urologist in the example above might claim that a circumcision amounts to cruel and degrading treatment under this article.

Article 4: Prohibition of slavery and Article 5: Right to liberty

In the early 1970s a Norwegian dentist who had compulsory duties in a remote part of the country brought about a case under article 4. He was not successful, and it is unlikely that a consultant bringing forward a case under this article or article 5 because of a compulsory contract would be successful, although it is interesting to consider our definitions of slavery and liberty.

These articles have particular implications for psychiatric practice. Lobbyists for the mentally ill usually claim that the individual rights of people with mental illness are invariably compromised by the interests of society at large. The Human Rights Act potentially allows psychiatric patients to challenge aspects of their care in relation to compulsory detention. However, the indication at the moment is that current clinical practice is not considered to be in contravention of these articles and practice is unlikely to change. In fact, as discussed in Case 12, the likelihood is that with the revisions of the Mental Health Act, the individual rights of patients with mental illness are likely to be more, rather than less compromised.

Article 6: Right to a fair trial

This article will have relevance to patients lodging complaints against doctors resulting in fitness-to-practise investigations. Along with the other recommendations resulting from the Shipman Inquiry (see Case 24), the Human Rights Act is likely to have a profound effect on the way in which the GMC conducts its processes.

Article 7: No retrospective crimes

In the example above, the urologist is protected by article 7, which claims that there are no retrospective crimes. However, this does not protect him in 20 years' time for circumcisions he performs now.

Article 8: Right to respect private and family life, home, and correspondence

The principles pertaining to medicine with regard to this article are largely those also covered by the Data Protection Act (discussed in Case 22). They may also cover the right of doctors to privacy with regard to intrusion from the media.

Article 9: Freedom of thought, conscience and religion, Article 10: Freedom of expression and right to information, and Article 11: Freedom of assembly and association

In relation to medicine, these articles might support the rights of whistle-blowers and would protect them from any adverse consequences resulting from expressing their views.

Article 12: Right to marry and found a family

This article has long been criticised as a questionable 'right'. It has potentially very serious consequences for the NHS if applied to the right of infertile couples to have children, or indeed those of post-menopausal women. This article has not yet been tested yet in this context.

Article 14: Right not to be discriminated against

The man who contacted the urologist in the example above could make a claim under article 14 on the basis of sex discrimination since female circumcision, also known as female genital mutilation, is already prohibited in the Prohibition of Female Circumcision Act 1985.

Summary

- The Human Rights Act puts the European Convention of Human Rights into UK law and makes society accountable to the individual.
- The most important articles relating to the medical profession are article 2 (the right to life) and article 3 (prohibition of torture and degrading treatment), although most of the other articles also have some relevance.

Reading

- Hewson B. Why the Human Rights Act matters to doctors. *BMJ* 2000; 321: 780–1.
- Hill G. Circumcision may disappear from medical practice. *BMJ* 2000; 321.
- Human Rights Act 1998. London: The Stationery Office, 1998.
- Macgregor-Morris R. Potential impact of the Human Rights Act on psychiatric practice: the best of British values? *BMJ* 2001; 322: 848–50.
- The Liberty Guide to Human Rights. www.yourrights.org.uk

Reference

1.   Horton R. Health and the Human Rights Act. *Lancet* 2000; 356: 9236.

Chapter Six

ETHICS AND LAW
IN PRACTICE

PRACTICAL ETHICS AND LAW AROUND THE WORLD

This chapter presents a range of cases from around the world, which describe the kind of ethical and legal dilemmas that have been encountered by doctors at all levels of training and in different specialties. The cases describe real scenarios, although patient data have been altered to ensure anonymity and protect confidentiality.

ETHICS AND LAW IN EMERGENCY MEDICINE

Case 1

Professor Peter Rosen – San Diego (CA), USA

The police brought a 32-year-old man into A&E. He had a gunshot wound of the right leg that was soft tissue only and apparently contained a bullet or bullet fragment. The bone was intact and this apparently had been a ricochet injury, according to the police. The patient wasn't telling anyone how the injury had been sustained.

Their report was that the patient had sustained the injury during a robbery that he was committing. It was alleged that he had shot and killed a convenience store clerk and had been shot by a police officer but had made a successful getaway. He was under arrest for suspicion of the robbery and murder. The police had a court order for the wound to be explored, and the bullet removed as evidence. The court order mandated exploration by any physician.

On physical examination, the patient had normal vital signs. There was a soft-tissue injury of the right calf that was neither infected nor extensive. A bullet fragment or bullet could not be palpated. An X-ray study of the leg revealed the bullet fragment, with intact bony structures. The issues in the case are the ethical concerns of the physician for the patient, versus the legal request of the police to help them acquire evidence to convict their suspect.

On medical grounds, there was no reason to explore the wound. Contrary to popular Hollywood tradition, there is no special need to remove bullet fragments, especially when there is no impending damage to nerve, artery or bone, and no sign of infection. The wound was actually healing nicely, and would do perfectly well with no medical interventions.

As a physician, my first ethical obligation is to the patient. It is not up to the physician to judge how the patient is injured, and there is no way I could produce a convincing argument that operating upon the leg would help this patient. There is no law that states that a prisoner has to accept medical treatment, and this patient wished to refuse all medical care. So, from a medical ethical point of view, there was no reason to treat the patient further. Legally, there are of course constraints upon any physician. In all jurisdictions with which I am familiar in the United States, there is a legal mandate to report wounds of violence, especially gunshot wounds. That wasn't an issue here because the police were aware of the wound and had been the ones to bring the patient to A&E.

The difficult ethical issue is whether the physician has to abide by the court order. While there may be a personal wish to support society over the individual, I found it impossible to justify performing an operation upon the patient that could not be deemed helpful in any way to the patient, even though it might easily have been deemed helpful to society at large.

I therefore refused to obey the court order. It seems to me that physicians have an ethical obligation to their profession that supersedes their ethical and, at times, legal obligation to their society. I have always felt revulsion at the physicians who acquiesced to the Austrian Empress's Law that prisoners be examined to assure that they were in good enough physical condition to withstand torture. There are numerous other societies who have had physicians place society ahead of the patient's needs, but I think this is an abandonment of the Hippocratic tradition that has stood up well for 2000 years.

The outcome of the case was that the patient was returned to jail, and other sources of evidence were found to enable his conviction. The police were not especially happy with my refusal, and I never talked to a judge, but I still feel strongly that this is a case where the physician's duty to the patient must take precedence over his duty to society.

Professor Peter Rosen, MD FACEP FACS
Professor of Clinical Medicine and Surgery and Director of Education
Department of Emergency Medicine
University of California
San Diego (CA), USA

Case 2

Dr Andrew Swain – Palmerston North, New Zealand

A 69-year-old man arrived by ambulance at A&E, accompanied by his family. His main complaint was of a significant haemoptysis one to two hours before. The history from the family indicated that the patient had been suffering from metastatic carcinoma of the lung that had spread to the liver and involved the oesophagus. He had been a long-standing heavy smoker. The patient's regular opioid medication had been administered that day. A first course of chemotherapy had just been completed.

Examination showed that the patient was severely centrally cyanosed and dyspnoeic. His respiratory rate was over 40 per minute. He was unable to answer questions and could only grunt. His oxygen saturation was only 85% on 12 litres per minute of oxygen administered through a reservoir mask. Rales were present throughout the chest. The patient's breathing progressively fatigued and his ventilation had to be maintained with a bag-valve mask. His blood pressure was elevated, there were no signs of cardiac failure and there was no fever. The ECG revealed sinus tachycardia only.

The prognosis was explained to the family. The daughter did not accept that death appeared imminent and she wanted all life-saving treatment to be administered. At this point, the hospital records arrived. The histology report confirmed small-cell carcinoma and the specialist considered that unless there was any prompt benefit from chemotherapy, the prognosis was abysmal.

At this point, the admitting physician attended and recommended high-dose antibiotics intravenously (piperacillin and gentamicin) despite the absence of any signs of septic shock and the main complaint of haemoptysis. The physician told the relatives that 'extremely strong medication' was being given and that this was the best that medicine could offer. Opioid was withheld to avoid further respiratory compromise. The patient died from respiratory failure in A&E approximately 15 minutes after the antibiotics had been administered, before he could be transferred to a ward.

What issues made it difficult?

- Lack of preparation and state of denial manifested by the relatives.
- False hope, given by the physician, that intravenous antibiotics would rectify the problem when the patient was drowning in haemoptysis fluid. The relatives were misled.
- Misuse of expensive antibiotics without clinical justification.
- Withholding of intravenous opioid which could have made the patient more comfortable pending his almost inevitable demise.

What did I do?

I acquiesced with this management plan as the physician had moved in to take over the patient's care and had spoken to the relatives. I did not want to cause any further distress.

What did I learn from it?

- To pursue the strength of my own convictions.
- To have managed the patient myself.
- To have advised the relatives that the prognosis was extremely bleak.
- To have supported ventilation and given adequate opioid analgesia while remaining with the patient until death; to have ensured that he was as comfortable as possible in the circumstances.
- To have withheld expensive antibiotics that were engendering false hope and were given without clinical justification.

Dr Andrew Swain, FRCS
Clinical Director, Emergency Department
Palmerston North Hospital
Palmerston North, New Zealand

Case 3

Dr Sophie Park – London, England

A 25-year-old man is brought into A&E by ambulance at 4 am. He has 35% second- and third-degree burns to his face, chest and upper limbs. On arrival in the department he is alert with a Glasgow Coma Scale (GCS) score of 15.

The ambulance crew report that this man was picked up from a sauna in a 'massage parlour'. The man had apparently fainted and fallen forwards onto the hot coals in the sauna. When asked if he had any family we could contact, the man stated he had no partner and did not want his parents to know his whereabouts. It soon became obvious this man required urgent intubation and had a significant risk of mortality. Before intubation, the lead nurse asked again for relatives' details which he refused. His friend arrived soon after he was intubated, having left the sauna before the accident. He revealed that the man did in fact have a girlfriend and a one-year-old child.

Difficult issues

- This man had significant burns to his face, arms and chest, which posed a significant threat to life.
- He required intubation due to the risk of airway oedema and for safe transfer.
- He would undoubtedly have, at best, severe burn scars for life.
- Due to his serious injuries, we would under normal circumstances contact relatives. We had to transfer him to another hospital for specialist burns care and were keen to let at least his mother know. Would this then leave his mother with the task of telling his girlfriend?
- Could we reveal the man's whereabouts without alluding to the cause of his injuries?

What did I do?

- First, this man's clinical situation was stabilised and arrangements made for a safe and urgent transfer.
- After discussion with my consultant, we asked the police to visit his mother's house and inform her that her son was very unwell and was to be transferred to a specialist hospital. The mechanism of injury was not explained.

What I learnt

- Issues surrounding consent can be very difficult, even if no clinical information is revealed other than the patient's presence in hospital.
- To allow an individual to make an informed decision, time is required to explain implications of the injury and subsequent decisions. In the emergency situation, this is not always possible and a decision thought to be in the patient's 'best interests' may have to be made.
- 'Value' reactions towards a patient's mechanism of injury should play no role in the clinical management of a patient, although objectivity may be very hard to practise.

Dr Sophie Park, MBChB DCH DFFP
GP Registrar
Caversham Practice
London, England

ETHICS AND LAW IN GENERAL PRACTICE

Case 1

Dr Emma Nelson – Dublin, Ireland

Ciara was 17 and attending a psychiatrist for help with anorexia nervosa. Her potassium levels had to be monitored due to a tendency for them to drop as a result of her vomiting. This, and support, were my main roles in her care as her GP. She always attended alone and phoned for her results and follow-up plan. On this occasion her potassium level was 3.2 mmol/l (normal range 3.5–5.0 mmol/l), requiring a prescription for supplements. However, it was her father who phoned, demanding to know the result. He was angry and quite aggressive, stating that she was legally a minor and that as her father he had a right to know.

The challenges

- Balancing an appreciation of his obvious distress and worry, and the need to protect Ciara and my relationship with her.
- Dealing with anger in the context of an ethical dilemma and the sense of immediacy and urgency that this angry telephone contact instilled in me.
- I was relatively inexperienced at the time and conscious of not being absolutely sure where I stood 'legally', though I felt sure about what was right ethically (or rather what 'felt right').
- I had no idea what Ciara's wishes would be in relation to me communicating with her father.

I explained the importance of confidentiality and trust, most particularly in this age group, and that I would like to give the result to Ciara directly as I had done previously. However, threatened with lawyers and the Medical Council, I finally crumbled and gave him the result and treatment needed. Luckily my relationship with her was unaffected. It turned out she had known he was calling and was unperturbed by this. It could have been very different, particularly with a condition that tends to wreak havoc in families and in teen adult relationships generally.

I now teach Teen Health to undergraduates and to GP registrars and always use this case to illustrate the importance of, and difficulties with, confidentiality in dealing with teenagers. Issues they invariably debate include:

- Does the previous level of involvement of the family in the illness and its care influence the management of the dilemma?

- Should a doctor be influenced by whether or not a teenager is living independently from parents?
- Does an insight into the relationship between a teenager and parents dictate in any way how such a situation is managed?
- Would the scenario be different if her potassium result had been 2.1mmol/l?
- Degrees of disclosure of information to a third party; is there such a thing as breaking confidentiality 'a bit'?

It also acts as a springboard to discussing dealing with confrontation, managing the needs of concerned relatives while preserving confidentiality, and pitfalls of communicating results. Students often ask what I did and appreciate honesty in my response. This critical incident has meant that I now clarify with teenagers who require investigation, at the outset, how they would wish me to proceed should such a situation arise.

Dr Emma Nelson
General Practitioner
Lecturer in General Practice, Royal College of Surgeons, Ireland
Programme Director, NAHB & RCSI General Practice Training Programme
Dublin, Ireland

Case 2

Dr Dhruv Mankad – Nasik, India

I was returning from a community health education session in a village at around midnight. On the way, a middle-aged man, Raghu rushed out waving his hands to stop our vehicle.

'Doctor please see my daughter,' Raghu said. Raghu's nine-year-old daughter, Nanda had had a high fever since the evening, with vomiting and neck rigidity. Clinically, it was acute meningitis.

'Let us go to the nearest hospital,' I advised. The nearest hospital was about an hour from her village. Raghu had returned from the market town by the last bus. There were no vehicles in the villages around. To my shock, her father said, 'No, please take us to a witch doctor because this is black magic.' I argued with him, and spoke to Nanda's mother and to the other villagers in an effort to convince the father that there was a danger to Nanda's life and that if hospitalised early, she could be saved.

The community believed the nearest referral hospital with all the facilities was a death den; this was because serious cases were always referred from villages in the district, and mortality was high. The tribe, which is dominant in the area, had several cultural beliefs different from the middle class. Education was poor and female literacy was only 7%.

Nanda's parents refused and the villagers kept silent, leaving the decision to Raghu. We waited but Raghu did not budge.

The dilemma

My ethical dilemma was whether or not I should move her to the hospital without her father's consent.

Though they had an irrational belief and faith in the witch doctor, I had the utmost respect for their cultural beliefs. I needed her father's consent because she was a minor and was semi-conscious. If I moved her without their consent and she died on the way, or at the hospital, my driver and I could have been accused of moving her without consent. This would be a risk with this particular community because we had only just initiated development work with them and our relationship was new. The community could also accuse her parents of not following their traditional faith. It would also have hurt their beliefs.

The people's livelihood was from single-crop agriculture with supplementary source of wage labour from the government. The cost of referring is high even if the government hospital is free, as there is the cost of prescribed medicine, and the loss of wages of two people accompanying the patient. Even if moved without consent, treating her would be a costly affair, which someone would have to bear. Moving her would mean a cost equivalent to three months' worth of income. However, not moving her held the risk of delay and of death.

What happened

An hour later, we finally left her after giving her an injection of penicillin, and a non-steroidal anti-inflammatory drug. We returned early next morning with adequate medicines to provide her treatment, even in the witch doctor's presence. We were told, however, that she had had a convulsion an hour earlier and had died. I felt sad and dejected.

What I learnt

I learned that in a life-threatening emergency, try to seek consent from the patient's relative with witnesses around. If no consent is given, do what you think is best to save her life after informing her relatives, no matter what the risk may be. In a developing country such as India, once a good rapport with the community had been established, it would have been possible for me to take Nanda to the hospital, even though her parents refused to consent. I believe, however, that in developed countries with good healthcare facilities, awareness about the individual's freedom is high, and the individual's beliefs and choices vary a great deal.

This case occurred in the 1980s, and since then we have started to train local community health workers to diagnose and treat simple illnesses, and diagnose and refer early seriously ill patients. As a development organisation, we also facilitated their pre-primary and primary education. The witch doctor is no longer functioning, even though there is no doctor at all except at the local primary health centre and at the referral hospital where they were earlier. Morbidity at the referral hospital remains high, but the education facilities have increased and the female literacy rate has doubled.

Dr Dhruv Mankad, MB BS
MacArthur Fellow, working on primary health care issues in rural areas
Nasik, India

Case 3

Professor Bill Shannon – Dublin, Ireland

One of the grown-up daughters of Mr Darcy (aged 86 and a widower living alone in Dublin's inner city), called me out to see her father in his home. He had recently been discharged from hospital, having had yet another dilation of his oesophagus performed to enable him to swallow his food. I was met by the caller, together with her sister and a brother in the kitchen of the patient's home and told, in no uncertain terms, that their father did not know of his true diagnosis of cancer of the oesophagus and that 'it would kill him if we were to tell him now'. I replied that while I would not go in to see him in his bedroom with any mission to tell him anything that he did not wish to know, neither would I lie to the patient if he were to ask me about the true diagnosis. The three family members accepted that I could not be expected to lie to their father, but were clearly apprehensive that I might upset the previously agreed conspiracy that the patient had a 'blockage of his gullet, often found in old people'.

What I found

The patient was a jolly 86-year-old man who said that he was fed up of going in and out of hospital to get the blockage of his gullet cleared and asked me if in fact his problem was due to 'old age', as he had lost some two stones in weight, or whether indeed the condition was 'something worse'? I replied by stating that I did not believe it could be explained by 'old age' and asked him how much he wished to know. His reply was that he suspected that it was something very serious and he would like to know the 'full story', particularly as he had heard his family discussing him in the nearby kitchen and felt that they were keeping something from him. I then told the patient that unfortunately his suspicions were correct, that he had cancer of the gullet and that surgery was not considered safe for him, in view of the extent of his disease and his other medical problems.

At this juncture, the old man sat bolt upright in bed and shook me by the hand, saying, 'Thank you doctor for telling me the truth . . . now they don't need to keep trying to protect me from it any longer. I've had a very good innings and only hope I get whatever treatment is needed as time goes on.' I assured him that he would and left to speak again to the family members assembled in the kitchen. I explained to them that their father had indeed asked me for the truth about his diagnosis, that I had told him the bare essentials and had assured him that the Hospice Home Care Team and myself would jointly take care of his medical needs from this time onwards. The family members expressed some concern about how he might be after this watershed visit, but also expressed relief that they no longer needed to keep the truth from him.

Lessons learnt from this case

- It is important for the family doctor to be sensitive to the family's concerns, but to remain focused on the patient's needs, which must take priority over those of the family.
- In most cases involving the breaking of bad news, the patient often suspects the worst, ie the true position, whereas the family often like to believe that they are protecting their loved one from the unspoken reality.
- Breaking bad news often allows a family to get closer to their loved one, than is otherwise possible if they try to engage in a long-term conspiracy of silence or avoidance.

What I might do differently next time

I would contact the hospital team involved in his care and suggest they might check with the patient as to how much he already knew and how much he wished to know about his condition. I would emphasise how important it was that both the hospital and family doctors spoke as 'one voice' when dealing with patients with serious illness and with their family members or closest carers in the community.

Professor Bill Shannon
Professor of General Practice
Royal College of Surgeons in Ireland
Dublin, Ireland

Case 4

Professor Valerie Wass – Manchester, England

As a GP you meet problems which can challenge loyalties between yourself, the patient and the community. Working in a community for many years leaves you in a very privileged position.

The practice was in a wealthy commuter zone of Greater London. The patient was a lady well known to me, as were her husband and her nine-year-old daughter, who attended the local primary school. Unfortunately they had had only the one daughter as the pregnancy had been complicated by a placenta accretia which had resulted in a very complicated hysterectomy and a massive blood loss requiring a transfusion of 54 pints of blood.

She presented suddenly on a Friday with a chest infection, insistent that she was really ill and needed a chest X-ray. I am afraid I was a little dismissive but when she had the X-ray on the Monday, it was clear it was indeed serious. She had *pneumonia*. Subsequently this was confirmed as secondary to AIDS.

In those days it was relatively common practice for GPs not to be informed when their patients had AIDS. Although she trusted me with the diagnosis, she was adamant that it should not be on her practice records and that I should not tell my partners or staff.

Her concern was that if the community knew (and many of the practice staff had children in the same school), her daughter would be shunned and treated as contagious – perhaps an irrational fear, but very real. Her hospital consultant was fully supportive of keeping the diagnosis confidential when I discussed the problem with him.

Every patient should be treated as potentially HIV-positive. However, my partners would have argued strongly that the medical records should be complete and, as they might well have to deal with associated problems, they should be aware of the diagnosis.

Rightly or wrongly, I respected her confidentiality, placing my loyalty to her before that to my practice team. The family were always most grateful. She died and I had frequent contact with her husband during his bereavement. Our mutual trust helped him come to terms with his grief. But was this the right decision? If my partners had known what I had done, I am sure they would have felt I had not trusted them to keep the information confidential, even though this was an essential part of our Code of Practice.

Professor Valerie Wass
Professor of Medical Education in the Community
Manchester University
Manchester, England

ETHICS AND LAW IN OCCUPATIONAL HEALTH

Dr Joan Saary – Toronto, Canada

The dilemma

Mr C is a 46-year-old accounting clerk who was referred for 'assessment of symptoms related to his workplace' by his family doctor. The chief complaint was fear of exposure to toxic substances believed to be the result of racial persecution by six other employees, one of whom was previously charged with assault. Mr C was absent from work on non-medical leave with pay because of these concerns.

The history was significant for the presence of other multiple fears of contamination. Physical examination revealed no evidence of any toxic syndrome. Mental status examination suggested possible depression. It was unclear whether his fears were based in reality, so he was referred for psychiatric assessment. This subsequently confirmed a delusional disorder requiring anti-psychotic medication.

At the first visit, Mr C presented an unsolicited letter addressed directly to the treating physician from his workplace manager which posed several questions regarding Mr C's medical condition and demanding the physician to respond.

The issue and resolution

The issue is one of disclosure, or entitlement to confidential information. In this case, the patient was referred by the family physician, not directly from the workplace. This was not a third-party examination. Because there was no consent form signed by the patient, a letter was sent to the manager stating only that Mr C did indeed have a medical condition preventing him from working, and for which treatment was being arranged. The specific questions would not be answered.

The key learning points

In third-party examinations it has been suggested that no patient–physician relationship exists, as the physician is working on behalf of the payer. Whoever pays for the examination, often an employer, owns the information and controls its release (depending on the jurisdiction), unlike an examination taking place in the medical system.

The letter from the workplace stated: 'it is the policy of [this workplace] to support employees whose illness . . . is affecting their ability to do their job . . .' So, Mr C's manager felt entitled to know 'what was going on'. Unless the patient consents to the release of such information, however, it remains confidential. In this case, the patient did eventually sign a consent form. Only information relevant to the planning of Mr C's return to work (such as functional limitations) was divulged. His diagnosis was kept confidential.

Dr Joan Saary, MD MSc FRCPC PhD(C)
Flight Surgeon
Occupational Medicine Consultant
CIHR Postgraduate Fellow
St. Michael's Hospital and University of Toronto, Toronto
Ontario, Canada

ETHICS AND LAW IN PSYCHIATRY

Dr Adrian Sutton – Manchester, England

Patrick was 11 years old when he had 'wanting to be dead feelings' again. Social Services and his school were extremely concerned about Patrick's emotional state and behaviour. Taken in conjunction with the suicidal thoughts and feelings, the information indicated a need for psychiatric assessment. In order to establish the level of acute risk and formulate a crisis management plan, an individual consultation was required. Two years earlier his father had reluctantly agreed to child psychiatric assessment and a limited intervention was possible. On this occasion Patrick's father refused to allow me to interview him.

I found myself in a dilemma. Given the risk of self-harm, should I advise Social Services to seek an Assessment Order under the Children Act to allow me to assess Patrick? However, he was fiercely loyal to his father so, if carried out with him knowing it was against his father's wishes, it could make it difficult to interpret what Patrick did or did not say. I told Patrick's father the nature of my concerns, and the possible steps open to me. He angrily told me that the judge would give the order anyway so I should just get on and see his son. I felt this would be compliance under duress, not 'informed consent', and that it could also precipitate suicidal behaviour. I was not prepared to proceed on that basis. I thought that Patrick's father's views might change, given his previous partial engagement with me.

Although I was uncomfortable about judging risk without actually seeing Patrick, my prior knowledge of him and the third-party information available left me thinking that he was unlikely to be at acute risk of attempting suicide and that the measures in place would protect him in the immediate situation. I decided to manage this risk while attempting to develop a co-operative approach with his father as this might have benefit in the long term. I did not immediately seek an Assessment Order and lived with the resultant anxiety and uncertainty.

Dr Adrian Sutton, BSc (Hons) MB BS FRCPsych UKCP
Consultant in Child & Family Psychiatry and Psychotherapy
Central Manchester Health Care Trust
Manchester, England

ETHICS AND LAW IN GENERAL MEDICINE

Case 1

Dr Alejandro Cragno – Buenos Aires, Argentina

Pedro is a 58-year-old man who was diagnosed with amyotrophic lateral sclerosis a few years ago. He lives in Argentina, is married and has three children of school age. Pedro is a philosophy professor but has not been in work for two years. He has been unable to find work since the economic collapse of his country that has caused widespread unemployment and social exclusion.

During the previous year, Pedro had been given the normal treatments, without improvement. The neurologist then informed him of a new medication that was in phase 4 of investigation. So far it seemed to be very effective, given the improvement that the published trials showed. The drug had been approved recently in the USA, but it had not yet been approved in Argentina. Nevertheless, the neurologist advised Pedro to ask his GP to prescribe it for him.

The GP in turn requested funding for the drug from the authorities of the Public Hospital. Despite the fact that Argentine pharmacology specialists and an eminent neurologist recognised the benefits of the drug and supported its use, the Public Hospital refused to obtain the drug. They asserted that the treatment had not been approved in Argentina, that there was little experience of the treatment; and fundamentally that the lack of funds available meant that it would not be economically viable.

Pedro despaired at this decision and appealed to the highest authorities of Argentina to help him to have a chance to live, as this drug may represent his only hope (though no guarantee) of survival. Ultimately the conflict was passed to the Hospital Bioethics Committee.

The dilemmas

Is it right that a society with serious economic problems prioritises funding of proven treatments over experimental ones? If a country does not have much money, should it stop testing new treatments and therefore stop medical research and progress?

In situations of economic deterioration, should doctors carefully select the information they give to patients regarding treatment options? Would it have been better if the neurologist had not told Pedro about the experimental drug if Pedro was unlikely to receive it?

The outcome

Pedro finally received the drug – the pharmaceutical company provided it to him for free.

What I learnt

Nowadays in my country we have serious economic problems; the health services are in crisis. We are often faced with situations where we know that the patients have more effective treatment options but the social insurance and the public services are unable to support these financially. If there is not enough money to offer the best treatment should we, as doctors, inform the patient about all the treatment options or only those that are available, even when the available treatments are not the best?

I believe the individual patient should know about all the options because there are some people who may be able to pay for treatment privately, if the social insurance or public services cannot pay. From the perspective of public services, the resources must be allocated according to priorities. The problem in my country is that there are no clear rules in the health system and as a consequence there are permanent conflicts between the managers and people.

Dr Alejandro Cragno, MD
Consultant Physician
Bahía Blanca Medical Association Hospital
Buenos Aires, Argentina

Case 2

Dr Anthony Toft – Edinburgh, Scotland

The dilemma

A 43-year-old woman presented with a three-month history of secondary amenorrhoea, heat intolerance and palpitations. Among various investigations, raised serum total thyroxine and low thyrotrophin concentrations were found, consistent with a diagnosis of hyperthyroidism.

She was referred for treatment with iodine[131] when clinical examination detected a small but diffusely enlarged thyroid and isotope studies were in keeping with a diagnosis of Graves' disease. She received 400 MBq iodine[131] and three weeks later was found to be 16 weeks' pregnant. The fetal thyroid could have been capable of concentrating radioiodine at the

255

time of therapy and there was, therefore, a risk of fetal hypothyroidism and neuropsychological disadvantage.

Difficult issues

Routine advice would be to recommend termination of pregnancy, particularly as this lady had had five previously successful pregnancies and this latest was unplanned. The patient refused the option of abortion. It later transpired that a pregnancy test had been requested as part of the initial investigations by the GP but had been wrongly reported to the patient as negative.

What was done

Monitoring was carried out by measuring thyroxine and thyrotrophin in fetal blood obtained by cordocentesis with a view to treatment with intra-amniotic thyroxine in the event of evidence of thyroid failure. Fortunately, fetal thyroid function was normal throughout pregnancy and at routine neonatal screening at five days. Subsequent development of the child has been normal.

What has been learnt

The issue is whether pregnancy testing should be routine in women of childbearing age before treatment with iodine[131]. It has been thought sufficient to provide written and verbal warnings to patients of the contra-indication to iodine[131] treatment if pregnant or planning pregnancy within four months. Whether this case, the first example of the inadvertent use of iodine[131] during pregnancy in our patient clinic in more than 5000 patients over the age of 35 years, should alter our policy is debatable. In the index patient, of course, pregnancy testing did not prevent the inappropriate use of radioactive iodine.

Dr Anthony Toft, CBE FRCP
Consultant Endocrinologist
Royal Infirmary
Edinburgh, Scotland

Case 3

Dr Shrilla Banerjee and Dr Peter Mills – London, England

The dilemma

Mrs GW was an 81-year-old widowed lady who lived independently and was accompanied by her married daughter. While out shopping, she collapsed and was brought to hospital via ambulance. She gave a history of breathlessness, followed by light-headedness, preceding the collapse. On examination, she had a blood pressure of 130/90 mmHg, and a loud ejection systolic murmur with a thrill in the aortic area. The murmur radiated to the carotid arteries.

Blood tests revealed renal dysfunction with a creatinine of 185 μmol/l, and a microcytic anaemia (haemoglobin 10.6 g/dl with a mean cell volume of 67 fl). All other blood tests were normal. Faecal occult bloods were positive and she gave a history of alteration of her bowel habit over the previous three months. Echocardiography confirmed aortic stenosis with a calculated Doppler gradient of 100 mmHg. She had severe aortic stenosis, mild renal failure and a microcytic anaemia possibly related to a large-bowel carcinoma.

Her daughter was concerned that her mother might lose her independence and was anxious that she should undergo cardiac surgery. What management should have been considered?

Difficult issues

This lady would benefit from aortic valve replacement (AVR). However, her co-morbidities put her at increased risk from the operation. The suggested mortality from AVR in the over-80s is 8.5%. (Kohl P, Kerzmann A, Lahaye L, et al. Cardiac surgery in octogenarians: peri-operative outcome and long-term results. *European Heart Journal* 2001; 22: 1235–43.) However, her renal dysfunction would increase her operative risk and may worsen during the post-operative period and require dialysis, possibly permanently. In addition, she would require further investigation of the anaemia and the change of bowel habit before cardiac surgery. She would also need to undergo coronary angiography to determine whether or not she had coexisting coronary disease that would further increase her operative risk.

The management

This patient went on to have the AVR after discussion with the consultant surgeon and cardiologist. She had a stormy post-operative course and required dialysis for two weeks, but was eventually discharged home well. Her anaemia was found to be related to an adenoma, which was removed at colonoscopy (covered with antibiotics). She will require surveillance colonoscopy at six-monthly intervals. She is now living independently once more.

The important learning point

The important point here is that as the patient was independent and mentally competent before her admission, the management options must be discussed with her. In the first instance she needed to be aware of the risks and benefits of any surgical intervention for aortic stenosis. She should have been allowed to judge whether she felt the procedure was appropriate and if she wished to be considered for surgery. While it is helpful to include her daughter in these discussions, informed consent is essential in this situation and she should meet the surgeon, so both may evaluate each other. The risks of not having the procedure done should also be defined, as there is a high risk of sudden death in these patients, if left untreated.

The final decision about surgery can only be made once the results of all relevant investigations are available. Do not assume that because her daughter wants the patient to have an operation, the patient herself will agree to major surgery.

Dr Shrilla Bannerjee, MB ChB MD MRCP
Specialist Registrar in Cardiology

Dr Peter Mills, BM BSc FRCP
Consultant Cardiologist

The Royal London Hospital
London, England

Case 4

Dr Kosta Calligeros – Edinburgh, Scotland

I was an intern in the third week of my first placement as a doctor and had been seconded to a small district hospital in rural Australia about 500 km from Sydney. I was just starting the weekend on-call and was handed over a 16-year-old female patient called Ruth who was suffering from multiple pulmonary emboli and infective endocarditis on a background of intravenous drug use. She had been admitted for intravenous antibiotics and anticoagulation therapy.

Ruth was of Aboriginal origin and lived in Sydney with her family. She was visiting extended family members in the town, and her mother was due to arrive the next morning from Sydney. The only person who had visited her in hospital was her boyfriend. However, he had been banned from the hospital earlier in the week on the suspicion that he had been supplying Ruth with drugs while on the ward.

The registrar also informed me that Ruth had self-discharged against medical advice the day before. However, she had returned later that night complaining of further pleuritic chest pains.

The next morning, the nurses paged me because Ruth was requesting a gate pass to visit her uncle. However, the registrar had explicitly told me she should only be permitted a gate pass in the company of her mother, so I told the nurses to keep her on the ward until I could attend – I was in the middle of seeing another patient who had shot herself in the foot by accident while trying to defend her son from a snake. By the time I arrived on Ruth's ward, half an hour later, one of the nurses had already signed her out on gate leave against my instructions.

Four hours later, Ruth returned and stated that she wanted to self-discharge. It was clear to me that she was under the influence of narcotics. Her mother had now arrived and insisted that I keep her daughter in hospital 'at any cost'. She was concerned that Ruth's life would be in danger if she left the hospital.

I tried to persuade Ruth to stay and she gave me numerous reasons why she needed to leave. Eventually she became angry and blurted out that she wanted to leave so she could take an overdose and kill herself.

At that point I consulted my registrar who advised me that she could be scheduled under the Mental Health Act because she was under the influence of drugs and because she had threatened to kill herself. He then said that he was going to the cinema with the consultant and that they would both be out of contact for two to three hours.

However, while I was doing this, Ruth attempted to abscond and security guards had been called to restrain her. The security guards stated that they were not keen to use physical force to restrain Ruth for any length of time unless we had explicit advice from the police that her detention was covered by the Mental Health Act.

Issues

- In Australia, a 16-year-old patient can consent to medical treatment, and they can also legally *refuse* medical treatment, regardless of the wishes of their parents. Therefore, it is not enough that Ruth's mother is consenting to her treatment. For Ruth to be treated, Ruth herself needed to consent to treatment.
- Although Ruth had threatened to commit suicide, I did not believe that she really intended to harm herself deliberately. I did not believe that she was mentally ill and, instead, it was more likely that she had made the comment on impulse. However, her threat gave me an excuse to keep her in hospital and administer treatment, which is what we as doctors believed was in her best interests.

What I did

I called the local police station for advice and two police constables came to the hospital to discuss the matter. Their view was that if Ruth absconded they would not take her into custody themselves for two reasons. The first was that there had been a recent Royal Commission investigating the high number of Aboriginal people dying in police custody, and they were therefore very reticent to become involved. Secondly, the hospital had no psychiatric services apart from a psychiatric nurse and was not registered as a designated place of safety in which people could be kept involuntarily under the Mental Health Act.

I sought advice from a psychiatrist in a larger town nearby. He advised me to control her with sedatives and anti-psychotics and to try to reason with her. He told me that Ruth could be kept at my hospital under the Mental Health Act (advice that conflicted with that of the police) until she was medically stable, and *could* then be transferred to his hospital for psychiatric treatment if necessary.

I also contacted the Guardianship Tribunal for legal advice. They advised that if Ruth refused to comply with treatment, they would conduct an emergency hearing to appoint her mother as legal guardian.

I discussed the issues with Ruth's mother who agreed that we should follow the psychiatrist's advice. The security guards physically restrained her while the nurses administered the intramuscular and intravenous medications. Once Ruth had been sedated pharmacologically, she agreed to stay in hospital for treatment. I then contacted my registrar to let him know what had happened.

The registrar and consultant both came to the hospital that evening and the consultant arranged for Ruth to be transferred to a Sydney hospital for treatment under the Cardiology and Infectious Diseases Teams.

What I learnt

This case illustrates the dilemma faced by doctors trying to act in a patient's best interests, while in the process compromising the patient's autonomy. If Ruth was mentally competent she had the right to refuse treatment, despite the fact she had a life-threatening illness.

I am still not entirely clear that any of my decisions changed the long-term outcome for Ruth but I did believe at the time that I was acting in her best interests.

The issues raised in this were very complex, resources were limited given the setting, and I believe the best course of action I took was to consult widely. I had been a doctor for only three weeks and thus any decisions I made individually were from a very light base of experience.

This case leaves many unresolved questions, including:

- Did the police's refusal to apprehend her make my orders to restrain her pharmacologically and physically illegal?
- How does a junior doctor reconcile conflicting information from more senior authorities on the management of such a situation?

Dr Kosta Calligeros, BCom BSc MB BS
SHO in Orthopaedic Surgery
Royal Infirmary
Edinburgh, Scotland

ETHICS AND LAW IN SPORTS MEDICINE

Dr Vassilis Lykomitros – Athens, Greece

The dilemma

A 21-year-old athlete was preparing to compete in the Olympic Games as a member of his national rowing team. During the mandatory pre-participation testing, a dysfunction in the cardiac conduction pathways was revealed. The athlete underwent further electrophysiological studies under sedation that showed an arrhythmic electric destabilisation.

The professor who conducted the test said that there was a slight chance that he could have a cardiac arrest during exertion or stress, stating as an example that he would never allow this athlete to pilot an aeroplane.

Despite the risk of suffering a fatal arrhythmia during intensive exercise, the athlete insisted that he should still be allowed to race in the Olympic Games. He argued that he had never experienced any symptoms before, despite much training and competition in previous years. He was otherwise completely healthy and his family history was also negative.

During multidisciplinary meetings with other colleagues, the idea of introducing a pacemaker into the athlete's body was discussed. This could, in theory, prevent episodes of arrhythmias from occurring. However, there was nothing in the international literature to show that this had been tried before, nor reports of any other solution which would allow him to continue his sporting activities.

What issues made it difficult?

- A laboratory test revealed a potential problem but clinically the athlete was asymptomatic, even during extreme exertion training for international competition.
- The athlete insisted that he be allowed to race – he was ready to put his life in danger because the Olympic Games were his dream and life ambition.
- All the Government authorities (Secretary of Sports, Rowing Federation, club, sports centre) refused to take responsibility for the ultimate decision, leaving it completely up to me as team doctor.

■ The Federation and Government refused to sanction the idea of introducing a pacemaker because it was too politically risky. They were worried about the negative press and public reaction which could result if it was discovered that athletes were being encouraged to risk their lives in order to represent the nation.

What I did

I decided to withdraw the athlete from the national team and the sport, but I could not persuade him to stop his private sporting life and continue a sedentary life in the future. This was very difficult for me because I know from personal experience that as a professional athlete you live for the excitement of competing, and the pride of representing your country. At international level, the sport takes over your life to the exclusion of nearly everything else, and you feel that if you cannot compete, your life is over.

What did I learn?

I learned that as an individual person you can do whatever you want with your life but as a member of a team you have to protect both yourself and the other team members.

Young people may be ready to give their lives for ideals but experienced people need to guide them by explaining facts. When you have the responsibility, sometimes you need to make hard decisions to protect human lives as the Hippocratic Oath states.

I regret that I hesitated about introducing a pacemaker in this athlete, which could have allowed him to compete and continue his career. However, this seemed a difficult road to take at the time because there was no international precedent. Several years later there are now papers from other countries describing the introduction of pacemakers in fine athletes in similar cases.

Dr Vassilis Lykomitros, MD
Orthopaedic Spinal Surgeon
Former Olympic athlete – Greek Rowing Team
Manager of Rowing, 2004 Olympic Games
Athens, Greece

ETHICS AND LAW IN PAEDIATRICS

Case 1

Dr Jamiu Busari – Curaçao, Netherlands Antilles

The dilemma

A 38-year-old woman delivered a baby girl prematurely. Shortly after birth, the baby was transfused with erythrocytes to treat an acute anaemia. The mother's obstetric history revealed three previous pregnancies, two of which resulted in spontaneous abortions and the third in a stillbirth. Due to her obstetric history and age, she had requested to see an obstetrician for antenatal screening for fetal congenital abnormalities. The obstetrician reassured her that despite her obstetric history, the pregnancy was not at risk. No antenatal screening tests had been performed.

In addition to the child's anaemia, dysmorphic physical features were found on examination. An ultrasound scan of the brain and computed tomography revealed extensive (grade IV) intracerebral bleeding. An echocardiogram of the heart revealed an open foramen ovale as the only abnormal finding.

The parents were so happy with this baby after all the previous (unfruitful) attempts at bearing a child. Sadly, they had to be informed of the baby's clinical condition and the poor prognosis. The decision was made to discontinue active medical intervention. Supportive care and comfort was provided until the baby's demise two weeks later.

What made the issues difficult?

■ Convincing the parents about our decision (based on medical grounds) to discontinue treatment. A conflict arose between the moral views on life and death, and my professional responsibility to act in the patient's best interest, which was to discontinue intensive treatment in this case. As a physician, the decision to abstain from active medical intervention was based on the child's poor prognosis and on the consensus from the collaboration with colleagues in allied disciplines. A second problem was informing the parents that intensive treatment was being discontinued, knowing how dear this pregnancy and child was to them.

- Convincing the parents (who were devout Christians) of the poor prognosis of their daughter's condition. Although the parents appeared to understand the severity of the situation from the medical point of view, they still held a strong belief that a miracle would happen and heal their daughter. It was difficult to convince them of the child's poor prognosis.
- Following the decision to abstain from further intensive medical care, the child received a second blood transfusion. This was because I believed that it was inhumane not to give blood when I knew the child was anaemic. In addition, computed tomography of the brain was repeated in order to re-assess the degree of the intracerebral haemorrhage.

What I did

- I ensured careful and detailed documentation of each meeting with the parents by both the nursing and medical staff.
- I acknowledged the parents' religious views and an attempt was made to have the parents meet the hospital's pastor for support.
- Upon my request, the clinical plan was re-examined and the medical orders clearly stated again. This was to avoid (more) confusion or sending conflicting messages to the parents that could falsely raise their hopes.

What I learnt

- A great degree of understanding, compassion and empathy should be exhibited in such circumstances.
- The views of the patient (in this case the parents) should be acknowledged, even when they are in conflict with medical findings. The intervention of allied services (eg pastoral) can be beneficial in such circumstances.
- There should be strict adherence to the medical plan after extensive multidisciplinary collaboration and consensus.

Dr Jamiu Busari, MD MHPE PhD
Consultant Paediatrician
St Elisabeth Hospital
Curaçao, Netherlands Antilles

Case 2

Professor Marcellina Mian – Toronto, Canada

Four-year-old Jennifer was wheelchair-bound because of severe weakness due to thalassaemia. She had a haemoglobin of 4mg/l. Her parents, Jehovah's Witnesses, had refused periodic transfusions and would not consent to splenectomy for Jennifer as the surgeon and anaesthetist would not do the surgery without a pre-operative transfusion to raise her haemoglobin into a safer range. The parents would allow the surgery if the physicians agreed to transfusing the child only if she decompensated intra-operatively. Through their network, the parents obtained the agreement from physicians at a smaller institution to do the surgery without transfusing Jennifer beforehand. Our dilemma was whether to allow her transfer or to notify the child protection authorities of the fact that Jennifer's life and wellbeing were being placed at increased risk.

The issues

■ The relative weight of spiritual and physical dictates in deciding on a child's best interest.
■ Defining the limits of parental right to choose the level of risk to which a child's life can be exposed.

Ontario child welfare law requires reporting of situations where a child's safety and wellbeing may be at risk. Accordingly, we reported the parents' plan to the authorities, giving the opinion that it would increase the child's risk of complications, including death, unacceptably (estimatedly from about 2% to 10%). After hearing from all concerned, the authorities allowed the surgery without elective transfusion. Jennifer did well.

The lesson learned was an appreciation of the subjectivity of risk-taking thresholds. Further, this case demonstrated the difficulty of promoting safe practice. The favourable resolution in this case did not affect the basic dilemma and is not likely to affect future practice. An unfavourable outcome, however, would have affected both health and social practice for the future in terms of placing greater emphasis on the need to safeguard the child's physical wellbeing.

Professor Marcellina Mian, MDCM FRCPC
Professor of Paediatrics
University of Toronto
Ontario, Canada

Case 3

Dr Hamish Wallace and Dr Elizabeth Morris – Edinburgh, Scotland

The dilemma

Emma had presented with acute lymphoblastic leukaemia two years ago when she was nine years old. Emma had acute lymphoblastic leukaemia that initially responded poorly to treatment. In addition, she had an abnormal chromosome pattern within the leukaemia cells, and for these two reasons she was deemed to be high-risk. She was switched to a more intensive induction therapy and eventually did achieve remission but, unfortunately, after 14 months of treatment she developed back pain and a limp.

As these were similar symptoms to those at presentation, her bone marrow was examined and this confirmed relapsed acute lymphoblastic leukaemia. There was no evidence of central nervous system disease at presentation or at relapse. During her 14 months of treatment there had been a number of admissions to hospital with side-effects of treatment, which the family had found extremely difficult and distressing.

The outlook for a young girl who relapses 14 months into treatment is extremely poor. Conventional practice in this situation is to give further intensive chemotherapy with a view to achieving a second stable bone marrow remission. This would be followed with total body irradiation and an allogeneic bone marrow transplant from either her sister or a matched unrelated donor.

The chances of achieving remission in this situation are at least 50%, but the chances of long-term cure of the disease after relapse while on chemotherapy are poor, and certainly less than 10%.

Further chemotherapy treatment would put her at high risk of developing infections, sore mouth and diarrhoea. Even if she should go into remission with intensive chemotherapy, the side-effects of total body irradiation would include a premature menopause with a life-long requirement for hormone replacement therapy and little or no chance, even with donated eggs, of carrying a pregnancy to term.

After discussion with the medical team, Emma's parents decided that their daughter had suffered enough and that she should not receive further chemotherapy. They were concerned about the side-effects of treatment and did not want to put Emma through a bone marrow transplant with all the short-, medium- and long-term side-effects that this was likely to entail. Emma's parents consulted widely, including their Jesuit priest, who agreed that they were making the correct decision, but the physician responsible for her care was unhappy with this.

The legal context

In the UK, a young person of 16 years or over is presumed to be capable of giving legally valid consent to treatment. A child or young person under 16 is presumed not to be capable of giving legally valid consent, but may be able to demonstrate that they are capable of doing so if they can show that they understand the implications of what they are consenting to. In the case of the child or young person under the age of 16 who is not deemed competent, the parents can give proxy consent to medical procedures which are considered to be 'in the best interests' of their child. It is the 'best interests' test for medical interventions, treatments and procedures that governs the right of parents to give proxy consent on behalf of their children for treatment.

Summary of ethical issues

In this case, the clinical team was faced with a ten-year-old girl who had leukaemia which had relapsed after 14 months of treatment, and whose parents had refused consent to further chemotherapy.

This is an unusual dilemma, which has serious ethical ramifications. Most parents in this situation would be happy to give consent to further treatment of their child, bearing in mind the chance of achieving a stable remission and the small (less than 10%) chance of achieving a cure. Would it be in her 'best interests' for Emma to have further treatment, with all the side-effects that may be entailed, or to move straight into a palliative care phase where the likelihood of death due to recurrent disease would only be a few weeks away?

Were Emma's parents in a sufficiently strong ethical position to deny their daughter further treatment, on the basis of the 'best interests' test? Was Emma, who was now ten years old, able to go against the wishes of her parents and give informed consent for further treatment? Would the medical and nursing teams be able to give Emma further treatment against her parents' wishes, believing this to be in Emma's best interests?

What actually happened?

It became clear that Emma herself had not been given the opportunity to decide whether she wanted further treatment or not. It is, of course, a natural reaction for parents to be protective of their children and very often they are keen for words like 'cancer' and 'leukaemia' to be avoided at all costs in discussions with the patients themselves.

Further discussion with Emma's parents allowed them to let Emma herself enter the debate. While it was clear that Emma had experienced significant side-effects during her first 14 months of treatment, she was not concerned about receiving further chemotherapy and even progressing towards a bone marrow transplant. Once she had become an active participant in the treatment decisions, it became quite clear that she wanted to have further treatment.

The opening up of the ethical debate to include the patient herself, although she was only ten years old (and certainly well below the legal age of consent), enabled her parents, the medical and nursing staff to come to a firm decision about further treatment that everybody felt happy with.

Emma received further intensive chemotherapy. She was hospitalised and required intravenous antibiotics, and during this period of time she was not particularly unwell. Five weeks into this second-line treatment, her bone marrow was examined and unfortunately did not show remission. In view of the fact that it was now extremely unlikely that a further block of treatment would achieve a stable remission and allow progression to bone marrow transplant, treatment was discontinued and she was discharged home for palliative care. Sadly, she died two weeks after going home.

Learning points

Young people under the age of 16 are not legally considered to be able to give valid consent to medical treatment, but are often able to understand the issues involved and give informed consent for further treatment if allowed to participate in the treatment discussions. Young patients should never be excluded from treatment discussions and they should be given the opportunity to become involved. It is essential that discussions take place in a language that they themselves can understand. In our experience, young people will often have strong views about their treatment, show great understanding of the issues, and give a lead to both their parents and the medical and nursing staff responsible for their care.

Dr Hamish Wallace, MD FRCPCH FRCP(Edin)
Consultant Paediatric Oncologist
Royal Hospital for Sick Children
Edinburgh, Scotland

Dr Elizabeth Morris, MB ChB MRCGP
General Practitioner
Edinburgh, Scotland

Case 4

Dr Christina Panteli – Thessaloniki, Greece

Several years ago, a seven-year-old girl called Maria arrived at A&E accompanied by her mother. She was referred to me, as the paediatric surgical registrar on-call, with soreness and itching of the external genitalia. The mother provided the information initially and described no history of trauma or any other previous illness or treatment. There was also no maternal gynaecological history to which the girl's symptoms could be attributed.

Maria seemed to be rather shy and unwilling to talk to me. She answered my questions with monosyllables that turned mostly to 'no' when it came to the topic of her complaint and any possible incident that she could link with her symptoms. Her mother looked quite relaxed, giving the impression that she considered the situation to be a minor problem.

On observation of the external genitalia, there was diffuse erythema without any perineal bruising, laceration or wound. There was no sign of a torn hymen but there was a whitish discharge on the vestibule which did not seem to be coming out of the vagina. Despite her age, I thought she may have vulvovaginitis and suggested we should examine samples of the discharge and urine. I started to discuss the procedure thoroughly with them.

While I was explaining the reason for the swab test, Maria's mother said (in the presence of her daughter) that Maria had occasionally complained to her about her father cuddling, touching and undressing her, while he undressed himself and 'played' with her. She had said that this was distressing and sometimes painful and that she did not particularly like it, but said that it was their 'little secret' which she was not supposed to confess to anyone. The mother was adamant that she did not believe her daughter because she was a child and therefore could not be trusted to tell the truth.

Suddenly the whole story was perfectly clear to me. I kept on suggesting laboratory testing, in order to buy some time with the mother, who I felt was not particularly keen on participating in the routine proceedings required in cases of abuse. I also suggested that we would liaise with the social workers and the psychologists so that the child could have an opportunity to talk about her alleged experience. Alternatively, I offered to admit the child in order to give them both some time to sort things out.

After our conversation, Maria's mother looked quite concerned and restless and although she agreed to have the tests done, she said she needed to consider the alternatives and would think about things while waiting for the results. In the meantime I talked to my consultant and to the forensic services and arranged an examination for a case of a suspected sexual abuse.

Half an hour later, Maria and her mother came back with a normal urine test. They had already made the decision to go home and could not even be persuaded to wait for the swab test result, despite my efforts. This decision, according to the hospital policy, required the mother to sign Maria out against medical advice and accept responsibility for taking her child home. I encouraged her to come back whenever she wanted to, and not to hesitate to contact me at any time, but she was impatient and was not willing to discuss the matter any longer.

Ethical issues that made this case difficult

■ Sexual abuse at such an early age without obvious signs can be suspected but not confirmed without a positive test for sperm.
■ A parent who either does not believe what the child says or who is in denial cannot be easily persuaded without evidence.
■ The child who reports any form of abuse is usually scared, embarrassed and unwilling to talk to a stranger, especially a 'figure of authority' such as a doctor.
■ Most doctors are not experienced in approaching a child in this kind of situation, which needs to be addressed very sensitively.

The standard policy for suspected abuse in Greece begins with referral of the alleged victim to the forensic doctor, who must perform a physical examination and order the essential laboratory tests. The usual situation is that the parent accompanying the child strongly demands immediate action. Occasionally the parent may need time, in which case the child is admitted so that they may stay in a safe environment until the standard procedure starts.

In the uncommon situation of the parent refusing consent and when the child's life is not in immediate danger, the only action the doctor can take is to report the case to the district attorney, who will take certain steps within the next few hours. In the meantime the child must be kept in the hospital despite the parent's opposition, and the only way to achieve this is through the intervention of the hospital security service until the police arrive. This process may even involve separation of child and parent. The doctor faces the dilemma of whether such a process would be in the best interests of a child who has possibly already suffered considerably.

What I did

Initially, abuse did not cross my mind at all, so I discussed all the possible causes of the symptoms. When I heard what Maria had previously declared to her mother, I mentioned abuse as a possible cause but deliberately avoided stating that this was definitely the case. I explained the procedures necessary to search for all possible causes for Maria's symptoms, including abuse.

When the mother told me they wanted to leave, I expressed my opposition. I explained again the possible consequences and the alternative ways of dealing with it.

At that point, the only option I had for keeping the child would have been to call the hospital security, the police and the district attorney in charge. I decided against this, believing this would cause Maria further anguish and distress.

The outcome

Two hours after Maria and her mother had left the hospital, I obtained the results, which were positive for sperm.

According to Greek law we should have reported the incident to the district attorney who would start legal proceedings. I had a long discussion with my consultant about the case. We believed that Maria's mother had been concerned about Maria's stories and came to the hospital seeking reassurance that Maria was lying. Not finding the reassurance she was looking for seemed to have disturbed her. The impression she gave me when she left was that she was probably going to take action, if she found further proof at home. Because I had explained all the options to her in dealing with abuse, including professional help, we agreed that it would be better for Maria if the matter could be dealt with within the family than going through a legal procedure.

They never showed up again, at least not in our department.

What I learnt from the case

In such cases child abuse must always be suspected.

Being a doctor does not provide you with the power to persuade other people to share your views and act in the way you believe is right.

Instinctively, I felt strongly for the child that evening. After a lot of thought and a couple of years I felt strongly for both of them. I faced an agonising dilemma and dealt with it in the way I believed was in Maria's best interests at the time. However, there are many unanswered questions: Did Maria's mother seek help again? Did she face the problem and take action? If yes, we made the right decision. However, if she decided to ignore and conceal what her child was going through, then our decision was utterly wrong.

Because we never found out if, and how, Maria's mother acted, I have been reconsidering how correct we were in our judgement. If we had ignored the extra emotional trauma Maria would go through in legal proceedings, we would have decided to report the possible abuse so that it could be dealt with. Instead, we chose to save her from that experience, but this deprived us of the satisfaction of feeling that something was being done. It is difficult to say whether or not we would make the same decision again – every case is unique and must be treated on an individual basis.

Dr Christina Panteli
Paediatric Surgeon and Honorary Specialist
G. Gennimatas Hospital
Thessaloniki, Greece

ETHICS AND LAW IN INTENSIVE CARE

Case 1

Dr Bob Taylor – Belfast, Northern Ireland

A nine-year-old boy presented with a severe brain injury as the result of an accident. Five days following his admission to a paediatric intensive care unit, appropriate tests confirmed brainstem death. Despite being given explanatory information by the medical and nursing staff, the child's father refused to permit the doctors to switch off the ventilator. Other options for management, including withdrawing or withholding treatment, were discussed by the doctors and the parents. These, however, were also refused.

Despite many hours of explanation, persuasion and argument, it proved impossible to obtain the approval of the father to discontinue ventilation. It was unclear whether the father had any legal rights in this matter. Again, several options were discussed, including stopping ventilation in any case. Despite the recognition that stopping ventilation at this stage, after brainstem death had been confirmed, would not result in criminal charges against the doctors, it appeared that the best option would be to continue ventilation until the situation could be resolved.

Good relations were maintained with both parents and it was accepted that they both had similar, if not equal, rights to consent for the minor but that the refusal of one parent outweighed the consent of the other. Therefore, with the agreement of both parents, social services were requested to seek wardship of the minor. This would clarify parental responsibility, ensure privacy and permit a court decision regarding withdrawal of artificial ventilation.

An emergency High Court sitting was arranged four days after formal brainstem tests had confirmed death. The trust applied to the court for wardship of the minor to be awarded to the local authority and to confirm that brainstem death equated to death. On the second court day the father contacted the doctors and requested that ventilation be terminated. The hospital trust therefore requested the court's permission to withdraw its application. This was granted, which effectively left the decision to discontinue ventilation back in the hands of the doctors and parents. The ventilator was switched off that same day, five days after the child had been declared brainstem-dead.

Dr Bob Taylor, MA MB FFARCSI
Consultant Paediatric Anaesthetist and Director of Paediatric Intensive Care,
Royal Belfast Hospital for Sick Children
Belfast, Northern Ireland

Case 2

Dr Stephen Child – Auckland, New Zealand

An 81-year-old lady was admitted to the medical ward with a 24-hour history of vomiting. She had no significant co-morbidity apart from mild osteoarthritis. She was subsequently found to be hypotensive and mildly hypoxic (oxygen saturation of 90%). Blood tests showed: platelets $72 \times 10^9/l$, mildly elevated liver function tests (LFTs) and a creatinine of 180 µmol/l with oliguria of 220 ml/24 hours. Our working diagnosis was one of sepsis (subsequently proved correct with positive (*Klebsiella pneumoniae*) blood cultures) with multi-organ failure and acute renal failure secondary to acute tubular necrosis (ATN).

We gave her fluids, inotropes, oxygen and antibiotics and asked our intensive care unit (ICU) to assess her for haemodynamic monitoring and potential dialysis or respiratory support if it became necessary. Our ICU replied that she was 'too sick' and that her poor prognosis precluded her admission to ICU.

We were then faced with the difficult dilemma of explaining to the family that their mother was too sick for us to 'try' to save her! I was furious. I knew that the literature for sepsis with three-organ failure and ATN concluded that she was facing a risk of 70% mortality but I did not accept that the ICU could protect their resources in this way and not accept a patient on these grounds.

To make the matter more interesting, the actual issue arose because we had also consulted the surgeons about her abdominal pain. They had responded that we should do a computed tomography (CT) scan of her abdomen – and if it showed a drainable collection, then they would see her but, if not, then she was not surgical. ICU initially said that they would take her if she went to theatre but would not if she didn't!

So what did we do?

First of all, I had an open discussion with my registrar, reviewing the medical facts and treatment options. I then expressed my opinion and we discussed our approach together to the family. We tried to get ICU to talk to the son directly but they refused, so my registrar eventually spoke to the son and outlined the likely futility of our actions anyway.

I spoke to the ICU consultant and flagged the case for our Quality Review. As I remained unsatisfied, I then presented this case to our hospital grand rounds and invited ICU to comment. The lecture theatre was packed with over 150 doctors and we had an excellent discussion on the topic. Essentially, ICU continued to defend its decision, based primarily on resources and all agreed to improve the communications between ICU and other hospital staff.

The woman did go into complete renal failure and was provided with palliative care from day 5. She died peacefully with her family at her side on day 11 of her hospital stay.

Dr Stephen Child, MD FRCP(C) FRACP
Consultant Physician and Director of Clinical Training
Auckland Hospital
Auckland, New Zealand

Case 3

Professor Graham Ramsay – Maastricht, The Netherlands
Dr Francesca Rubulotta and Professor Mitchell Levy – Providence, USA

Case description

A 79-year-old Caucasian woman presented initially with osteomyelitis in the lumbar spine (L1–L2) and received long-term intravenous antibiotics and oral opioids for lumbar back pain relief. The patient lived alone and at home. She developed shortness of breath, palpitations and left arm swelling and pain. After three days she presented in the emergency room where she was found to be hypoxic and to have atrial fibrillation. Past medical history included hypertension, diabetes mellitus, atrial fibrillation, atherosclerotic heart disease, and peripheral vascular disease.

The patient was transferred to the respiratory ICU, where she was sedated, intubated and ventilated, and a central line was placed via her left jugular vein. Her skin was cool and dry, and she had no fever or oedema. Her chest X-ray showed left lower lobe infiltrates and the ECG showed normal sinus rhythm with a rate of 140 bpm. She received medication for heart rate control, and the left central venous line was removed and cultured. The patient was successfully weaned off the ventilator but her ICU course was complicated by left subclavian-brachio-cephalic vein thrombosis and nosocomial pneumonia. Over the 12 hours after the extubation she developed hypotension, hyponatraemia and respiratory alkalosis. She was transferred to the medical ICU with the diagnosis of acute hypoxic respiratory failure and pneumonia in a patient with a high risk for pulmonary embolism. Her chest X-ray showed pulmonary infiltrates, highly suggestive, while the CT pulmonary angiography was negative, of pulmonary embolism. Seven days later, the patient was successfully weaned and transferred, alert and orientated, to a general ward.

She was probably discharged too early from the ICU and after 24 hours she was found to be lethargic, with an arterial pH of 7.19. She was re-intubated for hypercarbic respiratory failure and re-admitted to the ICU, where her systolic blood pressure dropped to 80 mmHg and white blood count rose to 31 × 10⁹/l. She developed a left knee effusion, right upper extremity cellulitis, right internal jugular line infection, and septic shock. Noradrenaline was started and continued for five days, to maintain normal blood pressure. The patient had a fever and a new chest X-ray showed extensive bilateral infiltrates, partial right middle and lower lobe collapse and atelectasis, with a possible malignant mass. The CT scan revealed changes in the posterior wall of a right intermediate bronchus. A bronchoscopy with broncho-alveolar lavage (BAL) and brushings of the right middle lobe were performed, revealing neither a clear source of pneumonia nor neoplastic cells. The vasopressor was gradually stopped, while bilirubin, urea, nitrate and creatinine continuously worsened from baseline levels. The arterial blood gases indicated significant metabolic acidosis and urine output decreased to less than 5 ml/hour.

Over the next three days she deteriorated, with pneumonia, sepsis, renal failure, increased pleural effusions, and pancytopenia. There was neither a living will, nor advance directives on the chart, nor much contact with the family. The patient was clearly incompetent to voice her wishes. Her relatives were contacted and the situation was explained to them. The two daughters participated together as patient's surrogate in the difficult process of decision-making. They realised the poor prognosis, and as they already had had a similar experience with their father, they knew, from earlier discussions at home, that their mother would not have prolonged this situation. They asked to have her made as comfortable as possible and the code status changed from Full Measures to Comfort Measures

Only (CMO). The patient was extubated and her breathing appeared laboured. To keep the patient comfortable, intravenous morphine was started at 5 mg/hour and titrated up to 7mg/hour. Her breathing became irregular and stopped. Her family remained quietly with her for a period after death was declared.

What can be learnt from this case?

Is palliative care fully adopted in intensive care units?

Despite advances in critical care medicine and in outcome research, death continues to be common in the ICU and less predictable than in the past decade.[1] In the case of this patient, the combination of multiple medical problems and the rapidly changing clinical status made predicting outcome a very difficult task. Many ICU patients die while still receiving aggressive interventions to extend life. A major challenge in hospital care is identifying better ways to cure illness while avoiding needless physical and emotional harm in terminal patients. The idea that palliative care should be detached from intensive care is no longer tenable. The main reason is that over the last century death has moved out of homes, and withholding or withdrawal of life support is becoming a common way of dying. An enormous amount of healthcare resources are delivered to dying patients,[2] and the considerable number of intensive interventions used before death is a troubling finding that critics argued might be inappropriate and inconsistent with patients' wishes. Currently, about 60% of Americans die in an acute care unit[3] but 90% of them would want to die at home.[4] Nearly half of all patients who die in the hospital are transferred to an ICU three days before death and the incidence of distress and discomfort seems to increase proportionally to aggressive care administration.

Should we gradually shift from aggressive therapies to palliative care or accept a sudden change from full code to CMO?

The ineffectiveness in determining the timing for the shift from primarily curative care to primarily palliative care is the main reason why the current patient received numerous invasive and expensive procedures just before death. The BAL performed the evening before withdrawing care, looking for lung carcinoma, might have been useful in making a decision. This invasive, low-risk procedure would not improve or change the patient's treatment. It is open to debate whether this or even other invasive examinations are necessary to make a correct decision in end-of-life scenarios. Numerous factors may limit the delivery of optimal palliative care in ICUs, such as the lack of sensitive or specific tools to assess patients' outcomes or inadequate training of professional care-givers. In the case of the present patient, we can state that uncertainty about the prognosis was the major barrier to optimal palliative care planning. The disease worsened extremely rapidly and left little time to shift gradually from cure to care measures. This situation is very common when treating patients with critical diseases, suggesting the need to link palliative care with critical care medicine. In modern ICUs one patient should either receive aggressive palliation or aggressive resuscitation.

Data suggests that there are unacceptable levels of suffering during ICU treatments, and several authors argue that much more could be done to relieve pain and anxiety, to respect personal dignity, and to provide opportunities for people to find meaning in life's conclusion.[5,6,7] Physicians should realise that there are many routine procedures that may cause unnecessary discomfort to hospitalised dying patients, such as daily laboratory tests, regular radio-graphic examinations, and frequent determination of vital signs. Distressing symptoms are underestimated by care-givers, even if they are associated with unfavourable outcomes such as a higher mortality.[8] There is no evidence that prevention of patient suffering would compromise aggressive efforts to prolong life, while the lack of pain and anxiety relief may limit the possibility of weaning and rehabilitating a patient. In one study authors showed that unrelieved, distressing symptoms are present even in an ICU, where their management is a major focus of attention.[6]

What would be the right time for the first meeting?

The lack of an appropriate relationship between the patient, her surrogates and the care-giver characterised the management of the present case. Communication with families in the intensive-care setting is difficult. Clinicians, counsellors, ethicists, researchers, and lawyers are researching this matter in an attempt to formulate guidance on how to hold meetings regarding life-sustaining issues.

Effective communication is a skill which requires several humanistic qualities, such as compassion, empathy and sensitivity. Both physicians and nurses working in an ICU need some general principles to be established regarding the patient–clinician relationship and trust. As stated Professor Levy has said: 'Unfortunately for our patients, the irony is that just because we see death all the time, we are not necessarily comfortable with it.'

Physicians cannot assume that patients or families will wish to plan death explicitly or will want to be actively involved in end-of-life care assessments. The result of one study showed that when the attending physician adequately communicates with families, more preferences are documented in the medical record and resource utilisation is decreased.[9] In the case of the present patient, ICU staff should have informed the family of the poor prognosis before the last admission. Establishing a relationship with patients and families is a new skill that ICU physicians have to accomplish in order to make appropriate therapeutic decisions. A national survey of 80% of US academic centres found that students, residents, and academic leaders evaluate themselves as inadequately prepared to provide compassionate end-of-life care.[10]

The implementation of a programme for training residents on ethical issues has an impact on patients' treatment and length of ICU stay for both survivors and non-survivors.[11] A significant proportion of people are not familiar with instruments such as living wills or durable powers of attorney. Fortunately, the surrogates in this case had had a previous experience and had discussed end-of-life preferences with their loved one before this hospitalisation. A meeting with the patient after her first extubation or before her discharge from the ICU, or even with her family, would have improved resource allocation and, above all, the patient's compassionate care.

What would the right number of meetings be and how much information should be provided?

One very important principle of compassionate care is that preferences and goals may change as an illness progresses. ICU patients often lose the capacity for decision-making during their hospitalisation, and surrogates do not always accurately reflect the right preferences. For this reason, ideally, patient-physician meetings should not be a single event. The severity of critical illnesses, however, does not leave enough time to meet patients or relatives more than once. Physicians need to be confident about what the patient's prognosis would be, before asking what 'he or she would like to receive as treatment'. This is a reasonable concept, knowing that the same patient may receive full aggressive intensive care from one healthcare provider and only comfort measures from another.[12]

May a previous family meeting shorten hospitalisation (the proxy had a similar experience in the past and knew the patient's wishes)?

Before holding a family meeting the physician should focus on what he or she would suggest as code status (resuscitation status). Dramatic differences in judgements were recorded in a large survey in Canada, in which physicians and nurses were asked about the appropriate level of care required for patients presented in different scenarios.[13] In the current literature the incidence of patients dying with full aggressive measures in place may range from 4% to 79%, while the incidence of withdrawing life-support ranges from 0 to 79%, with a high level of geographical variation. We may assume that the lack of an earlier meeting in the case presented would not necessarily have reduced the length of her ICU or hospital stay.

Should the physicians have re-admitted this patient to the medical ICU?

The possibility of re-admitting a patient depends on the specific ICU setting. Bed availability, for example, is a major factor in the use of intensive care in Spain, Portugal and the United Kingdom.

Was the last intubation strictly necessary?

The SUPPORT trial showed that a substantial majority of patients have not discussed preferences for life-sustaining treatment, even after 14 days of hospitalisation.[14] A large survey of several American thoracic critical care units[15] reported that 34% of physicians continued life-sustaining treatments despite patients' or surrogates' wishes, 25% of those who withheld or withdrew care did so without consent, and 14% did so without even the knowledge of patients or their surrogates. The percentage of patients with some kind of advance directive is about 10% in the United States, and those who had such directives are more likely to have documented orders or code status in their medical records. According to some authors, nearly 70% of patients have some restrictions on care before death.[16]

Conclusion

The dying process involves the healthcare system more and more and so physicians need to acquire end-of-life skills. The constant involvement of patients and surrogates in the decision-making process is a duty of modern ICU staff. Knowledge of the ongoing fusion between intensive care and palliative care is leading to new resource allocation and changing therapeutic goals.

Professor Graham Ramsay, MD PhD FRCS
Chairman of Intensive Care
University Hospital (Academisch Ziekenhuis)
Maastricht, The Netherlands

Dr Francesca Rubulotta, MD   **Professor Mitchell Levy, MD**
Research Fellow   **Chairman of Intensive Care**
Brown University   **Brown University**
Providence (RI), USA   **Providence (RI), USA**

References

1. Nelson JE, Danis M. End-life care in the intensive care unit: Where are we now? *Critical Care Medicine* 2001; 29: N2–N9.
2. Cher DJ, Lenert LA. Method of Medicare reimbursement and the rate of potentially ineffective care of critically ill patients. *JAMA* 2001; 278: 1001–7.
3. Field M, Cassel C. *Approaching death: improving care at the end of life*. Washington DC: National Academy Press, 1997.
4. Knowledge and Attitudes related to Hospice Care National Hospice Organization Survey. The Gallup Organization. Princeton: Gallup Organization, 1996.
5. Somogyi-Zalud E, Zhong Z, Lynn J, et al. Dying with acute respiratory failure or multiple organ system failure with sepsis. *Journal of the American Geriatric Society* 2000; 48: S140–S145.
6. Nelson JE, Meier DE, Oei EJ. The symptom experience of critically ill cancer patients receiving intensive care. *Critical Care Medicine* 2001.
7. Nelson JE, Meier DE. Palliative care in the intensive care unit. *Journal of Intensive Care Medicine* 1999; 14: 130–39, 189–99.
8. Chang VT, Thaler HT, Plyak HT. Quality of life and survival. *Cancer* 1998; 83: 173–9.
9. Dowdy MD, Robertson C, Bander JA. A study of proactive ethics consultation for critically and terminally ill patients with extended length of stay. *Critical Care Medicine* 1998; 26: 252–9.
10. Block SD, Sullivan AM. Attitudes about end of life care: a national cross sectional *study. J Palliat Med* 1998; 1: 347–55.
11. Holloran SD, Strakey GW, Burke PA. An educational intervention in the surgical intensive care unit to improve clinical decisions. *Surgery* 1995; 118: 294–9.

12. Kollef MH. Private attending physician status and the withdrawal of life-sustaining interventions in a medical intensive care unit population. *Critical Care Medicine* 1996; 24: 968–75.
13. Cook DJ, Guyatt HG, Jaeschke R. Determinants in Canadian health care workers of the decision to withdraw life support from the critically ill. *JAMA* 1995; 273: 703–9.
14. SUPPORT: A controlled trial to improve care for seriously ill hospitalized patients. *JAMA* 1995; 274: 1591–8.
15. Asch DA, Hansen-Flaschen J, Lanken R. Decisions to limit or continue life-sustaining treatment by critical care physicians in the United States: conflicts between physicians' practice and patients' wishes. *American Journal of Respiratory Critical Care Medicine* 1995; 151: 288–92.
16. Prendergast TJ, Claessen MT, Luce JM. A national survey of end-life care for critically ill patients. *American Journal of Respiratory Critical Care Medicine* 1998; 158: 1163–7.

ETHICS AND LAW IN SURGERY

Case 1

Dr Nermin Halkic and Professor Michel Gillet – Lausanne, Switzerland

A 36-year-old mother of two young children was admitted to the medical intensive care unit with a fulminant hepatitis of unknown origin. Consistent with this diagnosis, she had hepatic encephalopathy, a coagulopathy, and factor V of 42% (normal range 70%–140%).

Immunological tests revealed that she had chronic hepatitis B (HBV) in the reactivation phase. The reactivation was on a background of HIV with a viral load of 350,000 molecules/ml (>100,000/ml is very high), and a CD4 count of 180 × 10^6/l (normal range 700–1500 × 10^6/l). The general condition of the patient quickly worsened and the surgeon was faced with the decision of whether to carry out a liver transplant or not, knowing that this would be her only chance of survival.

The surgical team decided to go ahead and immediately carried out an orthotopic liver transplant. No major complications resulted and she has remained well since the operation, seven months ago.

This case re-ignited an already open discussion in all transplant centres, concerning organ transplantation in patients with HIV infection. It is not logical to transplant an organ into a patient in the terminal phase of HIV, for the same reasons as it is inappropriate to transplant an organ into a patient with chronic multi-metastatic hepatic carcinoma[1] because, despite the procedure, the prognosis is poor (life expectancy is only a few months). However, since the introduction of antiretroviral triple therapy, the survival of HIV patients has greatly improved. It is also now possible to control the incidence of opportunistic infections (the principal cause of death) in patients with chronic HIV.[1,2] Until now, only 40 cases of liver transplantation in HIV patients have been described in the literature. The mean survival time of these patients is 36 months, with a range of three months to 12 years.[3]

In view of the speed of development in antiretroviral therapy, we believe there is a place for transplantation in HIV-positive patients despite the current paucity of organs in Europe. We believe that transplant teams should learn from our American colleagues and completely revise their restrictive attitudes and discrimination policy against HIV patients who, in the coming years, could benefit from curative treatments.[1,4] HIV-positive patients who are otherwise well should be considered as normal patients with regard to all medical interventions, including organ transplantation.[5] In this particular case, the patient has survived and is doing well three years post-transplantation.

Dr Nermin Halkic, MD
Chef de Clinique

Professor Michel Gillet, MD
Chef du Service

Department of Surgery
University Hospital (Centre Hospitalier Universitaire Vaudois)
Lausanne, Switzerland

References

1. Halpern SD, Ubel PA, Caplan AL. Solid-organ transplantation in HIV-infected patients. *New England Journal of Medicine* 2002; 347: 284–7.
2. Roland M, Carlson L, Stock P. Solid organ transplantation in HIV-infected individuals. *AIDS Clinical Care* 2002; 14: 59–63.
3. Stock P, Roland M, Carlson L, et al. Solid organ transplantation in HIV-positive patients. *Transplantation Proceedings* 2001; 33: 3646–8.
4. Prachalias AA, Pozniak A, Taylor et al. Liver transplantation in adults coinfected with HIV. *Transplantation* 2001; 72: 1684–8.
5. Gow PJ, Pillay D, Mutimer D. Solid organ transplantation in patients with HIV infection. *Transplantation* 2001; 72: 177–81.

Case 2

Mr Jonathan Osborn – Chicago (IL), USA

A 96-year-old gentleman, Mr Smith, was referred by his GP to the urology clinic '. . . for discussion of a high prostate-specific antigen (PSA) result, and subsequent treatment . . .'.

One week previously he had been admitted under the physicians suffering from a myocardial infarction. He was a poorly controlled type 2 diabetic, and had been having crescendo angina for three weeks. He had also been taking warfarin for recurrent pulmonary emboli, and subsequently had not been offered primary coronary angioplasty. During that admission the house officer had ordered multiple blood tests, and had added a PSA test 'to be sure'.

In the discharge letter, the house officer commented that the PSA was 7.6 (local laboratory upper limit of normal for >70-year-old's is 6.5), and that the GP should refer to the urologists 'if indicated'.

On discharge, the patient received a copy of this discharge letter, and conducted searches on the Internet regarding PSA and prostate cancer. The patient therefore attended his GP appointment with six family members, grasping reams of Internet printouts regarding PSA and prostate cancer. Understandably, the GP felt pressurised to refer to the urologist.

At his urology appointment the patient was again accompanied by six relatives. Before I had even introduced myself, one of them said, 'We want you to do everything – we don't want him to be written off . . . We know he's got prostate cancer . . .' After this difficult opening, I succeeded in calming the situation down, took a history and performed a digital rectal examination, which revealed a 50-g benign-feeling prostate. It also became apparent that during his previous hospital admission he had developed a urinary tract infection (UTI), a condition that is known to increase the level of serum PSA. He had had no pre-morbid urinary symptoms. We discussed the fact that although a large number of men have prostate cancer, most of these men will die of their co-morbidities rather than the prostate cancer.

We had a frank discussion regarding the possible treatment modalities, in the event that he was diagnosed with prostate cancer. The patient was honest and told everyone that he did not want any curative treatment, because of the side-effects and risks. However, he would be keen on palliative therapies if the need arose.

His relatives were relieved because they were concerned that no one would listen to a 96-year-old, and wanted to support his right to choose his treatment. Once they realised that I was trying to act in the interests of the patient, they were much happier, and supported the patient in his decision.

We agreed that the patient was unlikely to have a significant prostate cancer, and that the mildly elevated PSA might, in fact, be due to the presence of a UTI. We also agreed that seeing the PSA fall to within normal limits would be reassuring. After three months his PSA was within normal limits, and all family members were delighted.

What issues made the case difficult?

- The assumption by the family that the patient had prostate cancer, and that I would refuse to treat the patient because of his age.
- Poor communication between the hospital, patient and relatives. The patient and his family were unaware why the test was ordered, and the implications of a positive test.

- PSA is an excellent monitoring tool for men with a proved history of prostate cancer to monitor disease progression. However, screening for prostate cancer using PSA is not widespread as PSA is elevated in a variety of conditions. Doctors and patients should be aware that many men over the age of 80 have prostate cancer, but that most will die from other medical conditions. This balance of risk and benefit is something that is difficult to convey and discuss.
- Having to provide information that might contradict what the patient has already been told by the GP.

What did I do?

I listened to the concerns of the patient and family, and painstakingly addressed each issue in turn. I was honest with the patient about the chance of a positive diagnosis, and the implications thereof. Faced with the information, the patient decided that he was not fit for curative therapy in the event of a diagnosis of prostate cancer. Furthermore, they decided that a biopsy was not indicated as curative therapy would not be considered, and that PSA monitoring would be appropriate. I had therefore attempted to educate the family so that they could come to an informed decision, rather than just telling them not to worry.

What did I learn from it?

- Not to underestimate the impact of doctors' words and actions upon patients and their families.
- The importance of discussing the reasons for ordering tests, and the implications of positive tests.
- Not to assume that an older man with a significant medical history would opt for non-curative therapy.

Mr Jonathan Osborn, MRCS
Urology Research Fellow
Midwest Urology Research Foundation
Chicago (IL), USA

Case 3

Mr Michael Carmont – Oswestry, England

An 89-year-old lady was admitted from a nursing home, having gone off her legs. At the time of admission she was confused, hypoxic and mildly tachycardic. She had a previous history of angina. She was apyrexial but had a leucocytosis and consolidation on her chest X-ray. Previously, she had mobilised with a frame around the home and interacted well with other residents.

She was admitted from A&E to a general medical admissions ward and given oxygen therapy and intravenous antibiotics.

Over the next couple of days she made little improvement and was intermittently confused. The nursing staff noted that she groaned as they moved her around the bed and that her left leg was externally rotated. An X-ray of her pelvis revealed a displaced intracapsular neck of femur fracture. The consultant physician explained to the family that she would need to have an operation on her hip and referred her to the on-call orthopaedic registrar.

Reviewing her that evening, the orthopaedic registrar noted that she was still confused, disorientated in time, place and person. The registrar explained the benefits of an operation in terms of analgesia. The patient then answered appropriately to the understanding of her problem and declined an operation in yes/no answers. She answered consistently, even upon repeated and varied questioning by both the registrar and the ward nurses, that she did not want an operation. Thus she refused to consent for an operation and was therefore kept comfortable in bed with analgesia prior to toilet and washing.

Next day, the consultant physician was surprised that the patient was still on his ward and called up the registrar on-call for that day to review the patient again. He insisted the patient needed an operation and said he was willing to sign a consent form saying that it was in the patient's best interests to have surgery. He reiterated this to the relatives, who were about to go on holiday abroad. On review, however, the patient still declined an operation.

The on-call orthopaedic consultant was called the following day and informed of the situation. He agreed that we could not operate on this lady as she was able to refuse consent for an operation, and recommended contacting the hospital's legal team. The case was discussed with the ethico-legal department and it was agreed that the patient was actively refusing an operation.

Over the next two weeks she gradually improved and became more orientated and less confused. When her relatives came back from their holiday, they found her awake and conversing appropriately. The family discussed the case and the patient decided that as she would not be likely to walk again without an operation, she consented to surgery. Two days post-hemi-arthroplasty insertion, she had a cerebrovascular accident and died.

Ethico-legal issues that made this case difficult

Communication between the medical and orthopaedic teams

Once a referral has been made to an on-call team within the hospital, subsequent communication about the patient should be directed towards the team caring for the patient rather than a new on-call team. This could result in two consultants making separate, conflicting decisions.

The explanation of the treatment options of surgery versus conservative treatment

There are a number of issues for discussion. Traditionally, patients with an intracapsular neck of femur fracture have a better outcome following surgery than with conservative management. Even if they never recover normal mobility, they have better sitting posture, allowing easier breathing. They are easier to nurse, making them less prone to pressure sores. However, with the improved awareness of the problems of recumbency, the improved medical management of co-morbidities and the risks associated with surgery, operative treatment may not necessarily be the best treatment for all patients.

So the consultant physician was correct in that for the majority of patients with this injury, their best interests lie in having operative treatment, but both treatment options must be explained to the patient. The orthopaedic team appreciated this and that the patient herself (not her physician) must consent to an operation unless she was incapable of making an autonomous decision.

The understanding of consent for an operation

Only doctors who are capable of performing a procedure should take consent for a procedure, although people who are specially trained in taking consent for a particular procedure may do so. Although the consultant physician may have understood what the operation involved, it is unlikely he could have actually performed a hip hemi-arthroplasty operation himself. Thus it would not have been considered appropriate for him to complete a consent form or to say that it was in the patient's best interests, despite his considerable experience in general medicine.

Patients may give written, verbal and non-verbal signals for consent or refusal for procedures. They may also be capable of consenting for some procedures and not others. In this case, the patient repeatedly indicated that she did not want to have an operation and so performing an operation would have been an assault.

The relatives going abroad on holiday

Procedures may be discussed with relatives if the patient agrees, although the relatives themselves cannot consent for a procedure to be performed. However, elderly people often feel vulnerable and may not be happy to consent for procedures without the presence of a relative.

What I learned

Involve the experts

In this situation where two experienced doctors from different specialties have differing opinions regarding ethico-legal problems, it is now more appropriate to seek help from the hospital's ethico-legal department. This enables consultants, expert in managing such problems, to be involved in the issue and reinforces that, as a junior doctor, you have acted responsibly.

Good documentation is essential

Knowing that the case was sensitive, a nurse was present during all discussions with the patient to act as a witness to her declining surgery. All discussions with the patient, relatives, medical and orthopaedic teams and the ethico-legal department were carefully documented in the patient's notes to ensure that everybody knew what had been discussed and the names of nursing staff present were also included in the notes as witnesses.

Mr Michael Carmont, MRCS
Specialist Registrar Orthopaedic Surgery
The Robert Jones & Agnes Hunt Orthopaedic and District Hospital
Oswestry, England

Case 4

Dr David Joseph – Sydney, Australia

A 67-year-old lady presented to A&E with a two-day history of abdominal distension, mild generalised abdominal pain, and vomiting. In addition, her bowels had not been opened for three days, with an absence of flatus for 48 hours.

Her past medical history included a laparoscopic cholecystectomy some years previously, hypertension, and a mild anxiety disorder.

The history was obtained with the assistance of the patient's daughter as English was not the patient's primary language and an interpreter was not immediately available.

Initial assessment revealed a dehydrated patient with a distended, mildly tender abdomen. There were no localising signs, and no evidence of rebound. The pulse rate was 86 bpm and regular, and the patient was normotensive. Radiological assessment included an erect chest X-ray, as well as erect and supine plain abdominal films. Multiple gas/fluid levels and a moderately dilated small bowel were found. The patient was managed with a nasogastric tube on low wall suction, and intravenous fluid therapy, and a provisional diagnosis of an adhesive small bowel obstruction was made.

Progress over the subsequent two days suggested some resolution, with flatus being passed, less distension in the abdomen, and no ongoing nausea. A limited intake of oral fluids was commenced.

However there was no further improvement, and a decision was made to perform a CT scan of the abdomen, looking for other causes of obstruction, given that adhesions from a laparoscopic cholecystectomy do not often cause obstruction.

Throughout the patient's stay in hospital, her daughter had been abrasive in her communications with the medical and nursing teams, and quite demanding regarding attention for her mother. This included requests for physiotherapy and advice from a hospital dietician, in the hope that through all this additional management guidance the daughter would be better able to manage her mother in the community post-discharge.

All this was to a point understandable except that she also was requesting that we limit the information provided to her mother, particularly regarding any setbacks in the patient's progress. This was requested on the basis of the patient's underlying anxiety and a desire not to cause undue distress.

An appointment with an interpreter was made and a multidisciplinary meeting held with the patient, the daughter, nursing staff, the dietician, physiotherapist, social worker, and myself. We wished to obtain further direct history from the patient, as well as explain to the patient our desire to perform additional tests and the possibility of an operation, depending on the tests results.

During this interview, some very relevant history was made available. This included a recent history (over a two-month period) of exertional angina, as well as an unplanned weight loss and change in bowel habit over the preceding three to four months. The patient's daughter was an active participant in this interview, and was noted at times to be interacting with the interpreter in their native language. The daughter asked why we wished to perform a CT scan, and with the newly available history, the possibility of a gastrointestinal malignancy was raised. Again the daughter wished to withhold this information from the patient, and may have had a role in doing this via her interactions with the interpreter.

The patient's subsequent progress was fortunately uneventful, with the CT scan demonstrating a mid-small-bowel, adhesive-type obstruction. A normal diet was restored over the ensuing few days. A cardiology assessment was made, and an out-patient appointment arranged for an exercise stress test and stress echocardiogram. Follow-up was arranged in the surgical clinic where a colonoscopy will be considered.

Relevant issues

A number of problems were identified in the management of this case:

- Failure to arrange prompt history-taking with the full use of an interpreter.
- Difficulty in addressing the daughter's concerns and, in so doing, losing the focus of the all-important doctor–patient relationship.
- Allowing the daughter to control the flow of information.

What I did

I allowed the daughter to function as the de-facto interpreter throughout the patient's stay in hospital. In hindsight, this restricted the flow of information both ways, and enabled the daughter to decide what was relevant to both her mother and to myself.

ETHICS AND LAW IN PRACTICE

What did I learn?

The importance of thorough history-taking and communication with the use of an interpreter. All too often and due to time constraints, clinicians accept family members and friends as interpreters. There are medically trained interpreters available, and every effort should be made to use them.

It is important to address the concerns of family members but the doctor–patient interaction takes precedence, and we should be aware of potential breaches of confidentiality when communicating with family members or using them as interpreters.

Dr David Joseph, MBBS FRACS
Surgical Superintendent
Royal Prince Alfred Hospital
Sydney, Australia

ETHICS AND LAW IN ANAESTHETICS

Dr Guy Routh, Cheltenham, England

As part of my clinical practice, I provide a service to the oncology department to insert long-term, indwelling central venous lines for the administration of chemotherapy. This procedure has a recognised morbidity and a small risk of mortality. Patients receiving cancer treatment often wish to discuss aspects of their treatment with all staff involved.

A 75-year-old man was booked onto my list for insertion of an indwelling line to enable administration of palliative chemotherapy for continuing management of his metastatic bowel tumour. He was free of symptoms and indicated that he was not certain why the procedure was being carried out. He lived alone in a small town some 15 miles from the hospital, had no means of transport other than limited public services, and was of limited intellect. His only income was his state pension. In my pre-operative assessment, it became clear that he was dreading the repeated visits to the hospital for his continuing care and had little under-standing of what the chemotherapy was expected to achieve for him. He was aware that he had cancer and thought that the treatment might provide a cure rather than simply delaying his deterioration. He had been counselled about the purpose and side-effects of chemotherapy but it was clear that he had not got a good grasp of its full implications.

In his terms, he was quite well and able to undertake all normal activities without hindrance. He had no close friends or relatives.

I discussed his case with the consultant oncologist who was managing his care and expressed my reservations about insertion of the indwelling catheter. The oncologist recognised that there was a problem but still felt it was appropriate and best practice to continue with chemotherapy.

Difficult issues

- Had this patient given genuinely informed consent for both insertion of the catheter and chemotherapy?
- What was my role in ensuring this patient received appropriate care?
- Would any change of approach confuse or distress the patient?
- If chemotherapy was not given, what was the alternative manage-ment?

What I did

I discussed the patient with the nursing staff looking after him and, as a result of this, telephoned his GP, who expressed some surprise that the patient was to receive chemotherapy as she felt that he was not really in a position to make a considered decision and was in generally good health at present. I then had further discussions with the oncologist, face to face rather than on the telephone, and we saw the patient together with a specialist oncology nurse. Following this meeting, it was agreed that we would neither insert the line nor administer chemotherapy at this stage but would arrange for the GP to keep the patient under review with an open appointment for specialist opinion if required.

The patient was not referred back for chemotherapy but when his condition deteriorated some six months later, he was managed at home by palliative care services for two months before being admitted to his local community hospital two days before his death.

Learning points

As an anaesthetist, you carry responsibilities for overall patient care over and above the provision of a 'technical' service. You are one of the clinicians managing the patient and should ensure that patients have been given sufficient information to make an autonomous decision about their care. An easy option would have been to simply proceed with insertion of the indwelling catheter but this would have been a failure of professional involvement with this patient. Although one consultant, in this case the oncologist, is in overall charge of the patient, all members of the team involved with his care have a responsibility to ensure that this is appropriate, taking into account clinical, social and other issues.

In this case, both the oncologist and the GP were unaware that insertion of long-term lines carries a significant risk and it is important that full information about such risks is available to all members of the team to ensure that correct advice is given to the patient.

It is important to avoid giving conflicting advice to the patient and, to achieve this, it is often better if those involved see the patient together.

Dr Guy Routh
Consultant in Intensive Care
Cheltenham General Hospital
Gloucestershire, England

APPENDIX

USEFUL ONLINE RESOURCES

British Medical Association
The BMA Ethics Committee contributes to major topical ethical debates by making influential reports and policy statements.
www.bma.org.uk – register login and go to 'Ethics' section.

Bulletin of Medical Ethics
Independent publication offering a source of current news and views on a range of issues in healthcare ethics, both in the UK and abroad.
www.bullmedeth.info

General Medical Council
All the guidance aimed to help you, but also the standards you will be accountable for upholding – essential reading!
www.gmc-uk.org – go to 'Ethical Guidance'.

Journal of Medical Ethics
One of the leading journals on medical ethics – some free papers available online; otherwise enter through your institution's database.
jme.bmjjournals.co.uk

Medical Defence Union (MDU)
Society that aims to protect doctors and provide legal guidance. The website details case studies which are useful learning resources.
www.the-mdu.com

Medical Protection Society (MPS)
Society that aims to protect doctors and provide legal guidance. The website details case studies which are useful learning resources.
www.mps.org.uk

Nuffield Council on Bioethics
Independent body with detailed examinations of ethical issues available free online.
www.nuffieldbioethics.org

World Medical Association
Online 71-page ethics manual with guidance on a wide range of ethical issues – and includes a list of further resources.
www.wma.net – go to 'Ethics Unit'.

CASE INDEX

SUBJECT INDEX